ICSS

INTERNATIONAL CONGRESS AND SYMPOSIUM SERIES 251

Editor-in-Chief: Lord Walton of Detchant

Appropriate Antibiotic Use

Edited by

Professor Don E Low MD FRCCP

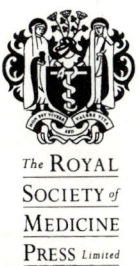

The ROYAL
SOCIETY of
MEDICINE
PRESS Limited

INTERNATIONAL CONGRESS AND SYMPOSIUM SERIES 251

© 2001 Royal Society of Medicine Press Ltd

1 Wimpole Street, London W1G 0AE, UK
207 E Westminster Road, Lake Forest, IL 60045, USA
http://www.rsm.ac.uk

Apart from any fair dealing for the purposes of research or private study, criticism or review, as permitted under the UK Copyright Designs and Patents Act, 1988, no part of this publication may be reproduced, stored or transmitted, in any form or by any means, without the prior permission in writing of the publishers or in the case of reprographic reproduction in accordance of the terms of licences issued by the Copyright Licensing Agency in the UK, or in accordance with the terms of licenses issued by the appropriate Reproduction Rights Organization outside the UK. Enquiries concerning reproduction outside the terms stated here should be sent to the publishers at the UK address printed on this page.

These proceedings are published by the Royal Society of Medicine Press Ltd with financial support from the sponsor LIBRA Initiative (Bayer AG). The contributors are responsible for the scientific content and for the views expressed, which are not necessarily those of the sponsor, of the editor of the series or of the volume, of the Royal Society of Medicine or of the Royal Society of Medicine Press Ltd. Distribution has been in accordance with the wishes of the sponsor but a copy is available to any fellow of the Society at a privileged price.

British Library Cataloguing in Publication Data
A catalogue record for this book is available from the British Library
ISBN 1-85315-496-2
ISSN 0142-2367

Phototypeset by Phoenix Photosetting, Chatham, Kent
Printed in Great Britain by Ebenezer Baylis, The Trinity Press, Worcester

INTERNATIONAL CONGRESS AND SYMPOSIUM SERIES 251

Guest Editor

Professor Don E. Low

Participants

Dr Antonio Anzueto
ASSOCIATE PROFESSOR OF MEDICINE, UNIVERSITY OF TEXAS — HSC AT SAN ANTONIO, 7400 MERTON MINTER BLVD, SAN ANTONIO, TX 78284, USA

Dr Joseph M. Blondeau
ROYAL UNIVERSITY HOSPITAL, 103 HOSPITAL DRIVE, SASKATOON, SASKATCHEWAN S7N 0Z8, CANADA

Dr G. Douglas Campbell
PROFESSOR, LSU MEDICAL CENTER, 1501 KINGS HIGHWAY, ROOM 6341, SHREVEPORT, LA 71103, USA

Dr Tim Clark
NATIONAL HEART & LUNG INSTITUTE, IMPERIAL COLLEGE, DOVEHOUSE STREET, LONDON SW3 6LY, UK

Ms Rita Kunz
ASSOCIATE DIRECTOR GLOBAL SCIENTIFIC AFFAIRS, BAYER AG, BUSINESS GROUP PHARMA, 42096 WUPPERTAL, GERMANY

Dr Ramanan Laxminarayan
FELLOW, ENERGY AND NATURAL RESOURCES DIVISION, RESOURCES FOR THE FUTURE, 1616 P ST NW, WASHINGTON, DC 20036, USA

Dr Steven Nelson
JOHN H SEABURY PROFESSOR OF MEDICINE, SCHOOL OF MEDICINE IN NEW ORLEANS, 1901 PERDIDO STREET, SUITE 3205, NEW ORLEANS, LA 70112-1393, USA

Dr Joseph A. Paladino
DIRECTOR OF CLINICAL OUTCOMES AND PHARMACOECONOMICS, STATE UNIVERSITY OF NEW YORK AT BUFFALO, CPL ASSOCIATES LLC, 3980 SHERIDAN DRIVE, AMHERST, NY 14226, USA

Dr Shelby D. Reed
PROGRAM IN PHARMACEUTICAL OUTCOMES RESEARCH AND POLICY, UNIVERSITY OF WASHINGTON, PO BOX 357630, SEATTLE, WA 98195-7630, USA

Dr Sean D. Sullivan
ASSOCIATE PROFESSOR, PROGRAM IN PHARMACEUTICAL OUTCOMES RESEARCH AND POLICY, UNIVERSITY OF WASHINGTON, PO BOX 357630, SEATTLE, WA 98195-7630, USA

INTERNATIONAL CONGRESS AND SYMPOSIUM SERIES 251

Dr Stephen H. Zinner
CHARLES S DAVIDSON PROFESSOR OF MEDICINE, HARVARD MEDICAL SCHOOL, CHAIR, DEPARTMENT OF MEDICINE, MOUNT AUBURN HOSPITAL, 330 MOUNT AUBURN STREET, CAMBRIDGE, MA 02138, USA

INTERNATIONAL CONGRESS AND SYMPOSIUM SERIES 251

Contents

iii
List of participants

vii
Preface
PROFESSOR DON LOW

ix
Introduction
DR TIM CLARK

1
Appropriate antibiotic use – past lessons provide future directions
DR JOSEPH M. BLONDEAU

11
International principles of appropriate antibiotic use
DR TIM CLARK

17
Minimizing the development of resistance with appropriate antibiotic use
DR STEPHEN H. ZINNER

21
Achieving maximum therapeutic effect through appropriate antibiotic selection and use
DR STEVEN NELSON

29
Select the most appropriate antibiotic first
DR G. DOUGLAS CAMPBELL

33
Criteria for appropriate antibiotic use in hospital and managed-care settings
DR ANTONIO ANZUETO

37
Reducing economic burden with appropriate antibiotic use
DR JOSEPH A. PALADINO

43
Socioeconomic issues related to antibiotic use
DR SHELBY D. REED, DR SEAN SULLIVAN & DR RAMANAN LAXMINARAYAN

49
The role of infectious agents in bronchitis
DR G. DOUGLAS CAMPBELL

57
The role of the pharmaceutical industry in fostering the appropriate use of antibiotics
MS RITA KUNZ

Preface

PROFESSOR DONALD E. LOW

CHIEF, TORONTO MEDICAL LABORATORIES AND MOUNT SINAI HOSPITAL
DEPARTMENT OF MICROBIOLOGY
HEAD, DIVISION OF MICROBIOLOGY, DEPARTMENT OF LABORATORY MEDICINE AND PATHOBIOLOGY, UNIVERSITY OF TORONTO, TORONTO, ONTARIO, CANADA

This publication is designed to introduce the concept of appropriate antibiotic therapy (AAT) and how it can minimize the emergence and dissemination of antimicrobial resistance while ensuring optimal patient management. It contains a series of papers written by key opinion leaders on various aspects of this approach to antimicrobial resistance control. Dr Joseph M Blondeau begins by asking what happens when good drugs are used inappropriately, Dr Stephen H Zinner discusses ways of minimizing the development of resistance through appropriate drug use, Dr Steven Nelson discusses how to achieve maximum therapeutic effect through appropriate drug use, and Drs Paladino, Sullivan *et al* discuss the socioeconomic issues, to name but a few. Between them, the following chapters paint a broad picture, illustrating the importance of AAT as a concept as well as detailing the practicalities of its implementation across the world.

The opinion leaders involved were brought together by LIBRA, a new international educational and scientific initiative conceived and developed by Bayer AG. LIBRA's stated aim is "to preserve antibiotic effectiveness for public protection" and, as the following pages reiterate, a key means of achieving this aim is by educating doctors, patients and policy makers to reduce the misuse, overuse and underuse of antimicrobials. It is hoped that LIBRA – the latin word for scale – will come to represent the balance that we need to achieve in antibiotic selection between the best choice for the patient and the best for the control of antimicrobial resistance.

Introduction

DR TIM CLARK

NATIONAL HEART & LUNG INSTITUTE, IMPERIAL COLLEGE, DOVEHOUSE STREET, LONDON SW3 6LY, UK

This publication is designed to introduce the concept of appropriate antibiotic therapy (AAT) use and a series of papers by key opinion leaders on various aspects of this topic. The papers are:

- Appropriate antibiotic use — past lessons provide future directions — Dr Joseph M. Blondeau
- International principles of appropriate antibiotic use — Dr Tim Clark
- Minimizing the development of resistance with appropriate antibiotic use — Dr Stephen H. Zinner
- Achieving maximum therapeutic effect through appropriate antibiotic selection and use — Dr Steven Nelson
- Select the most appropriate antibiotic first — Dr G. Douglas Campbell
- Criteria for appropriate antibiotic use in hospital and managed-care settings — Dr Antonio Anzueto
- Reducing economic burden with appropriate antibiotic use — Dr Joseph A. Paladino
- Socioeconomic issues related to antibiotic use — Dr Shelby Reed *et al.*
- The role of infectious agents in bronchitis — Dr G. Douglas Campbell.

The following sections paint a broad picture of the importance of AAT and its practical application in various regions of the world.

Appropriate antibiotic use – past lessons provide future directions

DR JOSEPH M. BLONDEAU

ROYAL UNIVERSITY HOSPITAL, 103 HOSPITAL DRIVE, SASKATOON, SASKATCHEWAN S7N 078, CANADA

The discovery of compounds with antimicrobial activity was a major advancement in medicine and patient care. These compounds provided doctors with an adjunct therapy to the patients' own immune system — the principal and perhaps best defence for fighting infectious diseases. The negative consequences of antimicrobial use were quickly realized, however, when bacterial strains showed elevated minimal inhibitory concentrations (MICs) to antimicrobials, and therapy failed. This initial observation should have been an immediate warning of the vulnerability of antimicrobial agents in the face of the enormous potential of bacterial pathogens for mutation and replication. Unfortunately, it was not, and new agents being introduced from either natural or synthetic sources continued to be used following established practices, so, unsurprisingly, the consequences have remained the same too.

Antimicrobial resistance is now a pandemic

Unfortunately, antimicrobial resistance is now a global pandemic[1-6]. Figure 1 shows the mechanisms of antimicrobial resistance, the major classes of antimicrobial agents affected, and the genetic structures in the bacterial cell where resistance genes can be located. Sporadic reports of antimicrobial resistance for various pathogens are increasingly common and such potentially dangerous trends should be monitored carefully. Equally, a small number of bacterial strains can be resistant to an antibiotic despite large clinical trials indicating considerable sensitivity (very low MICs) to the antibiotic. Due to the replicative capabilities of the bacteria, there is more chance that small numbers of resistant bacteria, present in suceptible bacterial populations will be selected or that new mutations will be selected, so in today's environment guaranteed efficacy is unlikely for most pathogen–antibiotic combinations.

Broadly, antimicrobial resistance can be based on three major mechanisms[7]: decreased uptake, altered membrane permeability and efflux, which all affect the total intracellular concentration of the antimicrobial agent. Put simply, if the concentration of the compound in the bacterial cell is insufficient then the organism is rendered resistant. Enzymatic destruction results in physical modification of the antimicrobial structure so that it is no longer biologically active – the target/binding sites are altered which causes a decrease in binding affinity of the compound with the target, sometimes to the point where the compound cannot bind at all. This either creates an increase in the amount of antimicrobial required to inhibit the pathogen, or full resistance. Additional complicating factors in antimicrobial resistance are the observations that bacteria may possess more than one resistance mechanism, and that resistance genes may be located on transferable genetic elements such as plasmids and transposons, which facilitate the spread of resistance between bacteria. Table 1 shows antimicrobial resistance in some common pathogens. The most serious outcome of antimicrobial resistance is clinical failure. Consequences of clinical failure include prolonged symptoms, clinical deterioration, hospitalization (possibly in intensive care) or prolonged hospitalization (accompanied by potentially increased mortality), the need for aggressive intervention (ie surgery), additional drug costs, decreased quality of life, reduced productivity and/or absenteeism from work.

Table 1 Antimicrobial resistance in selected pathogens

Organism / Agents affected	β-lactams	Macrolides/azalides	Clindamycin	Vancomycin	Fluoroquinolones	TMP/SMX	Older fluoroquinolones**	Tetracyclines	Aminoglycosides	Ampicillin/amoxicillin	Penicillin
Gram positive											
Staphylococcus aureus	•	•	•	•	•						
Enterococci spp	•	•		•	•						
Streptococcus pneumoniae	•	•	•			•	•	•			•
Gram negative											
Enterobacteriaceae	•				•			•			
Nonfermentative bacilli	•				•			•			
Haemophilus influenzae							•			•	
Moraxella catarrhalis							•			•	
Neisseria spp										•	

** ciprofloxacin, levofloxacin/ofloxacin, norfloxacin.

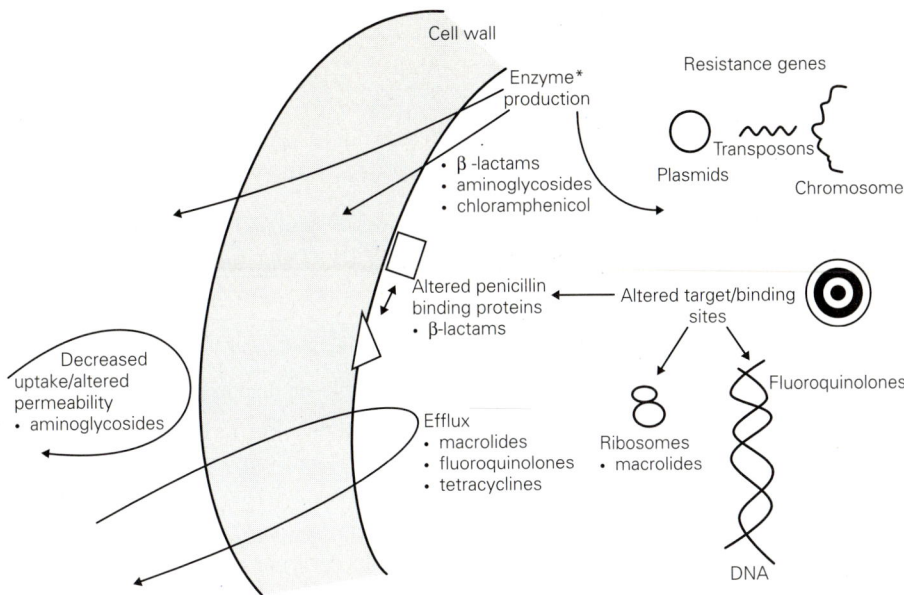

Figure 1
The mechanisms of antimicrobial resistance. *β-lactamase – penicillins, cephalosporins, extended spectrum b-lactamases; aminoglycoside inactivating enzymes, chloramphenicol acetylase, dehydrofolate reductase
Modified from Blondeau 2000[12]

Overuse of antimicrobials is, at least partly, responsible

Factors contributing to the emergence of antimicrobial-resistant pathogens are shown in Table 2. Most experts agree that overuse of antimicrobials contributes to the emergence of antimicrobial resistance, simply due to the selective pressure of antimicrobial use. Clinical trial data are doing a great disservice to these agents. Clinical trials are designed to show equivalency between compounds, and the time periods chosen for taking comparative measurements (ie 10 days) are not always likely to emphasise existing differences. Results which reveal differences between antimicrobials can help physicians select the most appropriate drug. Clinical trials tend to exclude patients who have a pathogen which is resistant to the study drug. There is a tendency to investigate the lowest dose that is effective at the least frequent dosing interval which could be seen to be desirable from a marketing perspective, but rather less than ideal from a microbiological or pharmacological view.

The right agent at the right dose and dosing interval and for the right duration can achieve both a favourable clinical outcome and prevent the selection of resistance. Wise *et al* cited that

Table 2 *Factors contributing to increased antimicrobial resistance*

- Overuse of antimicrobials — human, veterinary, agricultural
- Low dosages
- Improper dosing frequency
- Extended duration of therapy
- Prophylactic use
- Non-human use (veterinary)
- Clinical trials excluding patients with resistant pathogens
- Clinical trials which focus solely on clinical outcomes

20–50% of antimicrobial use in humans was questionable or inappropriate, compared to 40–80% used in agriculture[8]. Low and Scheld[9] suggested that doctors overprescribe antibiotics for the following reasons:

- patient expectations
- insufficient time with patients to discuss why an antibiotic is not needed
- concern over misdiagnosis and the fear that a patient with a bacterial infection does not receive an antibiotic and consequently deteriorates.

Impact of resistance on community-acquired respiratory tract pathogens

Considerable evidence has accompanied the dramatic increase in antimicrobial resistance of community-acquired respiratory tract pathogens to commonly used antimicrobials. The principal culprits include *Moraxella catarrhalis*, *Haemophilus influenzae* and *Streptococcus pneumoniae*. For *M. catarrhalis*, the principal mechanism of resistance is via the β-lactamase enzyme, which destroys β-lactam antibiotics. Data suggest that 85–100% of all *M. catarrhalis* isolates globally are ampicillin/amoxicillin resistant; however, resistance to amoxicillin/clavulanic acid, extended spectrum macrolides, cephalosporins and fluoroquinolones remains low at ≤3%[6]. Some data suggest that resistance to trimethoprim/sulphamethoxazole (TMP/SMX) is also changing — recent US data indicated that 16–51% of *M. catarrhalis* isolates were not susceptible to TMP/SMX at breakpoint (breakpoint is the drug concentration below which an organism is considered susceptible, and above which it is considered resistant).

For *H. influenzae*, the principal mechanism of resistance is via β-lactamase production. Table 3 shows selected antimicrobial resistance in *H. influenzae* from a global perspective. There are global problems with ampicillin resistance and tetracycline resistance has also been documented. More importantly, considerable resistance to TMP/SMX has been observed in many parts of the world, without generating particular concern in the medical community. For

Table 3 *Antimicrobial resistance in* Haemophilus influenzae

	Amp	Resistance (%) Tet	TMP/SMX
North America	26–42	1–2	3–32
South America	10	?	?
Europe	2–35	10	2–35
Middle East	19–28	8	29
Africa	7	?	12–17
Asia-Pacific	35–37	5	7–53

Blondeau and Tillotson[18]. Amp = ampicillin; Tet = tetracyclin; TMP/SMX = trimethoprim/sulphamethoxazole; ? = data not available.

example, Blondeau et al.[10] recently reported that 15 to 28 of 566 *H. influenzae* isolates taken from Canadian medical centres were TMP/SMX resistant, most commonly amongst organisms producing β-lactamase enzyme. In vitro susceptibility results suggest that, however, second- (cefuroxime>cefprozil>ceflacor) or third-generation cephalosporins and fluoroquinolones retain high levels of activity against *H. influenzae*.

Penicillin-resistant *S. pneumoniae* (PRSP) will probably present one of our greatest therapeutic dilemmas in the foreseeable future. During the 1990s, there was a dramatic increase in the incidence of PRSP in a number of different geographical areas around the world. While resistance to penicillin is worrying, perhaps an even greater concern is the coincidental cross-resistance to other drugs, such as β-lactam/cephalosporin agents, macrolides, tetracyclines and TMP/SMX. Cross-resistance to vancomycin and fluoroquinolones has not yet become a problem, but there are early warning signs of an increase in ciprofloxacin- and levofloxacin-resistant pneumococci in Canada[10]. It is true that the use of ciprofloxacin for treating pneumococcal pneumonia has been controversial due to the agent's borderline activity and treatment failures have been reported for ciprofloxacin, and also for levofloxacin and other classes of antimicrobials.

Fluoroquinolones are designed to target one of two intracellular targets: older fluoroquinolones target topoisomerase type IV, whereas, newer fluoroquinolones preferentially target DNA gyrase, in addition to having significant activity against topoisomerase type IV. Cross-resistance to the newer fluoroquinolones gatifloxacin, gemifloxacin and moxifloxacin will, therefore, probably occur at a slower rate.

Table 4 summarizes selected antimicrobial resistance in *S. pneumoniae* globally. The levels of penicillin resistance vary from one region to another, but resistance is prevalent in all major geographical areas. Significant resistance to the macrolides, tetracycline and TMP/SMX is also prevalent in *S. pneumoniae*.

Table 4 *Antimicrobial resistance in* Streptococcus pneumoniae

	Pen	Resistance (%)* Macro	Tet	TMP/SMX
North America	22–50	10–30	2–8	10–32
South America	20–24	3–6	32–45	0–35
Europe	7–42	5–51	0–29	8–57
Middle East	55	4	11	22
Africa	35–39	6	7–23	25
Asia-Pacific	6–65	0–90	82	70–87

*Includes intermediate and high level
Blondeau and Tillotson[6]. Pen = penicillin; Macro = macrolides; Tet = tetracyclines; TMP/SMX = trimethoprim/sulphamethoxazole.

An inpatient or outpatient problem?

In the 1980s, the selection and spread of antimicrobial resistance was felt to be primarily an internal problem for hospitals. Patients admitted to hospitals acquired resistant organisms and then carried them into the community. By the 1990s, patients were still acquiring resistant organisms in hospitals, but more importantly, resistant pathogens were occurring firstly in the community or in long-term care facilities, and were then brought into hospitals. As a result, in the 1990s, the prevalence of antimicrobial resistance became a significant issue for primary care prescribers treating community-acquired infections.

Archibald *et al* observed that the prevalence of antimicrobial resistance varies between inpatients and outpatients[11]. They compared resistance rates in 1997 for particular antimicrobial–pathogen combinations taken from inpatients and outpatients in the US (Table 5) and their analysis highlighted the following:

Table 5 *Resistance rates: sentinel antimicrobial–pathogen combinations for inpatients versus outpatients (p<0.01 unless marked)*

Agent/pathogen	Inpatients (%)	Outpatients (%)
Methicillin/Staph CoN	49.0	35.9
Methicillin/*S. aureus*	32.7	14.6
Ceftazidime/*E. cloacae*	26.0	11.9
Imipenem/*P. aeruginosa*	12.0	6.5
Ceftazidime/*P. aeruginosa*	7.8	4.0
Vancomycin/*Enterococcus* spp	6.3	1.4
Ciprofloxacin/*E. coli*	0.5	0.7*
Ceftazidime/*E. coli*	0.2	0.5*

From Archibald *et al*[11]; Staph CoN = coagulase negative staphylococci; *= non-significant.

- *Escherichia coli* resistance rates to all drugs except ciprofloxacin and ceftazidime were significantly higher in the inpatient population. However, *Staphylococcus aureus* and *Enterobacter cloacae* resistance rates were significant (14.6% methicillin-resistant and 11.9% ceftazidime-resistant respectively) in the inpatient and outpatient populations respectively.
- The increasing resistance of *Enterococcus* to vancomycin is further eroding the efficacy of a key agent active against enterococcal infections.
- The movement of antimicrobial-resistant pathogens is two-way: from inpatients into the community and from outpatients in the community into healthcare facilities.
- Antimicrobial protocols must take the prevalence of antimicrobial resistance into account.
- The implementation of strategies to combat high levels of resistance may be difficult.

One specific concern over the use of extended spectrum β-lactam agents (cefotaxime/ceftriaxone, ceftazidime) — important compounds for treating nosocomial infections — is the increasing prevalence of gram-negative bacteria which are producing extended spectrum β-lactamase enzymes. Such organisms which produce extended spectrum β-lactamase enzyme have been shown to increase morbidity and mortality and may be difficult to detect in clinical microbiology laboratories. Interested readers are referred to a recent comprehensive review[12,17].

Antimicrobial concentration is relevant

Negri *et al* provided evidence to suggest that it is not just exposure to, but concentration of, antimicrobial agent that is important[13]. When a mixed population of *S. pneumoniae* with various penicillin susceptibilities (MICs of 0.015, 0.5, 1 and 2 µg/ml) was exposed to low concentrations of β-lactam antibiotics, the susceptible strains were eliminated, but low-level (MIC values between 0.1 and 1 µg/ml) and high-level (MIC values above 2 µg/ml) resistant strains increased. When the same mixed population was exposed to higher concentrations of β-lactam antibiotics, however, the number of resistant bacteria was reduced because low-level resistant strains were also eradicated.

Investigations with moxifloxacin by Dong *et al* showed that a typical bacterial population contains organisms of varying sensitivities to a range of antibiotics[14]. This work demonstrated that when large numbers of bacterial cells (10^{10} cfu/ml) were tested using fluoroquinolones, those with resistant phenotypes could be detected among the 'susceptible' population. Such resistant bacteria could not be detected using previous susceptibility techniques relying on an inoculum of 10^5 cfu/ml. When fluoroquinolones were tested against a large number of cells, the concentration required to inhibit the most resistant first-step mutants (carrying one resistance-enhancing mutation) was called the mutant prevention concentration (MPC). The MPC represents a dosing threshold above which mutants should only rarely be selected[15].

A novel method of measuring antibiotic resistance

A series of subsequent reports[15] from the author's laboratory demonstrates the potential value of MPC in calculating the appropriate use of antimicrobials. When three fluoroquinolones were tested against 111 clinical isolates of *S. pneumoniae*, differences were found between compounds in terms of their MPC_{90} values (Table 6), ie the drug concentration required to prevent the selection of resistant mutants for 90% of the strains tested[14].

Table 6 Fluoroquinolone potency based on provisional MPC

Fluoroquinolone	MPC_{90}	MIC_{90}	C_{max}*	Bronchial tissue level
Gatifloxacin	4	0.5	3.7 (400 mg)	4.2
Levofloxacin	16	1	5.2 (500 mg)	7.0
Moxifloxacin	2	0.25	4.5 (400 mg)	5.8

*All dosed once-daily

When the MPC data are compared with the pharmacological data it becomes clear that the accepted current dosages are probably insufficient for levofloxacin to prevent the selection of resistant mutants. Other studies suggest the same concern for other common pathogens. For example, Blondeau and Tillotson[6] showed that ciprofloxacin was 2–24 times more active than levofloxacin in preventing the selection of resistant *Pseudomonas aeruginosa* mutants when both compounds were rated by MPC. Ongoing work with non-fluoroquinolone agents suggests that other antimicrobials can also be compared by MPC.

Strategies for antimicrobial use — the past versus the future

Past strategies for the use of antimicrobial agents have essentially recommended:

- that narrow-spectrum agents be used
- that agents be used at the minimum doses possible based on clinical trial data
- that antibiotics be used for unnecessarily long periods of treatment.

The net result of such strategies has been the emergence of antimicrobial resistance. Rather than dwelling on the past, the immediate question needs to be 'Are there any strategies that may be available to reverse, halt or slow the emergence of antimicrobial-resistant pathogens?'

because the answer to this question appears to be 'Yes'. Based on recent work from the author's laboratory using the MPC, an alternative strategy may involve:

- using more potent (not necessarily broader-spectrum) antimicrobial agents at the outset
- using more appropriate (perhaps higher) doses and more appropriate (more frequent) dosing intervals
- using antimicrobials for appropriate (possibly shorter) durations.

Conclusions

Taken together, the future use and preservation of antimicrobial agents appears contingent upon the following points:

- Appropriate use of antimicrobials; reduced overuse.
- An understanding of antimicrobial resistance and epidemiology.
- Prescriber understanding of clinical, pharmacological and microbiological variables.
- An appreciation that the current supply of agents is exhaustible.

Or, as two of our worthy colleagues have put it: "Our hopes of stemming the tide of antimicrobial resistance in North America depend not only on the success of these initiations, but also on the efforts of individual physicians"[9]. "Parochial approaches are, therefore, doomed to failure"[8].

References

1. Craig WA. The future — can we learn from the past? *Diagn Microbiol Infect Dis* 1997; **27**: 49–53.
2. Gold HS, Mollering RC. Antimicrobial drug resistance. *N Engl J Med* 1996; **335**: 1445–53.
3. Jones RN. Can antimicrobial activity be sustained? An appraisal of orally administered drugs used for respiratory tract infections. *Diagn Microbiol Infect Dis* 1997; **27**: 21–8.
4. Kunin CM. Resistance to antimicrobial drugs — a worldwide calamity. *Ann Intern Med* 1993; **118**: 557–61.
5. Levy SB. The challenge of antibiotic resistance. *Sci Am* 1998; **278(3)**:46-53.
6. Blondeau JM, Tillotson GS. Antimicrobial susceptibility patterns of respiratory pathogens — a global perspective. *Semin Respir Infect* 2000; **15**: 195–207.
7. Blondeau JM, Jensen B. Coping strategies for antibiotic resistance. *Can J Cont Med Educ* 1998; **10**: 47–61.
8. Wise R, Hart T, Cars O et al. Antimicrobial resistance is a major threat to public health. *BMJ* 1998; **317**: 609–10.
9. Low DE, Scheld WM. Strategies for stemming the tide of antimicrobial resistance. *JAMA* 1998; **279**: 394–5.
10. Chen DK, McGeer A, De Azavedo JC, Low, DE. Decreased susceptibility of *Streptococcus pneumoniae* to fluoroquinolones in Canada. Canadian Bacterial Surveillance Network. *N Engl J Med* 1999; **341**: 233–9.
11. Archibald L, Phillips L, Monnet D et al. Antimicrobial resistance in isolates from inpatients and outpatients in the United States: increasing importance of the intensive care unit. *Clin Infect Dis* 1997; **24**: 211–5.
12. Blondeau JM. Community-acquired respiratory tract pathogens and increasing antimicrobial resistance. *J Infect Dis Pharmacotherapy* 2000; **4**: 1–28.

13 Negri MC, Morosini MI, Loza E, Banquero F. In vitro selective antibiotic concentrations of β-lactams for penicillin-resistant *Streptococcus pneumoniae* populations. *Antimicrob Agents Chemother* 1994; **38**: 122–5.

14 Dong Y, Zhao X, Domagala J, Drlica K. Effect of fluoroquinolone concentration on selection of resistant mutants of Mycobacterium bovis BCG and Staphylococcus aureus. *Antimicrob Agents Chemother* 1999; **43**: 1756–8.

15 Blondeau JM, Zhao X, Hansen G, Drlica K. Mutant prevention concentrations of fluoroquinolones for clinical isolates of Streptococcus pneumoniae. *Antimicrob Agents Chemother* 2001; **45**: 433–8.

16 Hansen G, Zhao X, Drlica K, Blondeau JM. Mutant prevention concentration (MPC) of ciprofloxacin (C) and levofloxacin (L) against urinary isolates of *Pseudomonas aeruginosa* (PA). In: *22nd International Congress of Chemotherapy*. Amsterdam; 2001: 27.

17 Blondeau JM. Extended spectrum beta-lactamases (ESBL). *Semin Resp Infect* 2001: (In press).

International principles of appropriate antibiotic use

DR TIM CLARK

NATIONAL HEART & LUNG INSTITUTE, IMPERIAL COLLEGE, DOVEHOUSE STREET, LONDON SW3 6LY, UK

There has been a very significant reduction in morbidity and mortality associated with the use of antibiotics since they were first introduced, but, there has also been a concomitant rise in resistance among pathogens over the past 50 years. Moreover, antibiotics are sometimes associated with adverse events, and their use can account for a significant proportion of the cost of treatment of some conditions. To ensure optimal use of antibiotics, doctors should use the most appropriate antibiotic to stop each infection in each patient. This strategy of appropriate antibiotic therapy (AAT) can be achieved by careful attention to the type of infecting microbe or microbes, local resistance patterns and the socioeconomic resources of the medical facility and community in which the patient is being treated.

Benefits of AAT

There are numerous clinical, social and economic benefits to be realized from the use of rapidly acting, optimally effective, yet safe, antimicrobial regimens (see Paladino, pg 37). If infecting pathogens are eradicated more rapidly, the patient should recover more quickly and return to a normal lifestyle. The less time a patient is in a morbid condition, the fewer healthcare resources that person will require, and the sooner he or she can become a productive member of society again. Furthermore, eradicated bacteria are redundant and thus not able to develop and spread resistance.

Achieving maximum therapeutic effect through AAT

Ideally, the exact strain of the microbe that is causing the infection is identified before any antibiotic is dispensed. However, most therapy is, through necessity, empirical. In other words, the most appropriate antibiotic is selected according to the doctor's knowledge of the pharmacokinetics (PK), pharmacodynamics (PD) and resistance of the available drugs.

The area under the inhibitory time curve (AUIC) may be the most clinically important measure of a drug's efficacy. The AUIC is the ratio of the area under the curve (AUC) to the minimum inhibitory concentration (MIC) — combining the factors of drug concentration, microbial susceptibility and time. The AUIC correlates well with the efficacy of the tetracyclines, fluoroquinolones and aminoglycosides, as well as vancomycin, azithromycin, quinupristin and dalfopristin[1]. The doctor is more likely to achieve a clinical cure if an AUIC above 250 is reached (see Paladino, pg 37). The use of agents that have a significant post-antibiotic effect (PAE) may also be advisable. Other considerations in antibiotic selection include the ability of the drug to reach the site of infection, as well as the age and health of the patient (see Nelson, pg 21). Some key opinion leaders have created systems to stratify patients in order to recommend the most appropriate therapy[2].

Avoiding antimicrobial resistance with AAT

Low dosing and prolonged administration at sub-MIC levels — especially among agents lacking a significant PAE — are associated with an increased risk of developing antibiotic resistance (see Campbell, pg 29). With respect to the optimal use of specific antibiotics to minimize resistance, it has been observed that the use of an agent that kills bacteria very quickly and that stays above the pathogen(s)'s MIC for a long time should not only ensure that the infecting pathogens are eradicated, but that the incidence of development of resistance will also be reduced dramatically (see Campbell, pg 29). Rapid killing will not only reduce the development of resistance but could decrease patient mortality during the first five days of infection.

Numerous reports have established that resistant bacteria frequently emerge in hospital settings (see Anzueto, pg 33). The use of empirical antibiotic therapy and broad-spectrum antimicrobial agents in hospitals may increase the effect of selective pressure. For example, between 1989 and 1994, vancomycin resistance in hospital-acquired enterococci rose from 0–14%. Various gram-negative rods such as *Enterobacteriaceae* and *Pseudomonas* spp are now becoming resistant to third-generation cephalosporins and quinolones, while methicillin-resistant *Staphylococcus aureus* is now endemic in many healthcare institutions.

The imposition of arranged barriers to improper prescribing has had some success in reducing the overuse of antibiotics. In response to an outbreak of vancomycin-resistant enterococcal (VRE) infections, one hospital in Virginia, US, changed its computerized ordering system for dealing with vancomycin orders[3]. Before a prescription for vancomycin could be issued, the prescribing doctor was required to choose one of a list of approved indications as established by the Hospital Infection Control Practice Advisory Committee (HICPAC) of the Centers for Disease Control and Prevention (CDC). Paediatric, surgical and medical services all participated in the new system. In addition, the hospital instituted other changes, including better handwashing and isolation precautions, improved disinfection, and the use of surveillance cultures from high-risk patients. Within three months, orders for vancomycin fell from 103 g per 1,000 patient days to 54 g per 1,000 patient days, a reduction of 47%. The hospital's average expenditure for vancomycin fell from $13,103 per month for the five months before the outbreak, to $6,212 per month for the year following. Over the same period, the level of inappropriate orders had fallen from 61% to 30%. Most significantly, the incidence of VRE acquisition fell significantly, without any increase in other forms of infection attributable to the limitation of vancomycin use.

A teaching hospital in Utah, US, installed a sophisticated computerized system of managing antimicrobial use[4]. Designed to address antibiotic prescribing for empirical, therapeutic and prophylactic surgical purposes, the system's decision support programs provided immediate information based on consensus practice guidelines which the staff had previously established. After seven years, the average duration of antibiotic use after surgery, the incidence of antibiotic-associated adverse drug events, and mortality, all fell significantly, with the cost per patient of antibiotic treatment reduced by over 60% (see Anzueto, pg 33).

National responses to resistance

The Scandinavian countries have led the way in establishing programmes to combat resistance (see Zinner, pg 17). In Finland, a nationwide campaign was used to reduce the prescription of macrolides to combat the emergence of erythromycin-resistant group A streptococci[5]. As a result, the level of macrolide use fell from 2.40 doses per day per 1000 people in 1991 to 1.38 in 1992. The concomitant reduction in erythromycin-resistant isolates fell from 19.8% to 12.9% between 1993 and 1995. Another example is the Swedish Strategic Programme for the Rational Use of Antimicrobial Agents and Surveillance of Resistance (STRAMA)[6]. After the initiation of this programme in 1992, the frequency of penicillin-resistant *Streptococcus pneumoniae* (PRSP) stabilized at approximately 3% by 1997.

Ensuring optimal socioeconomic benefits from AAT

Other practical steps can be taken by countries around the world to ensure that the full benefits of AAT are achieved. These include (see Reed, pg 43):

- Sourcing timely, accurate, geographically specific and site-specific surveillance information regarding antibiotic resistance patterns to inform policy makers, doctors and researchers.
- Funding epidemiological research to explore the relationship between changes in the prevalence of antibiotic resistance and changes in the level of antibiotic prescribing. (Necessary for economic evaluations of the cost of resistance.)
- Using educational efforts to narrow the communication gap between doctor and caregiver/patient perceptions about antibiotic overuse. (Improving the appropriateness of use.)
- Educating patients about the risks associated with misuse of antibiotics. (Motivating responsible use.)
- Targeting relevant and personalized educational efforts towards doctors about their patterns of antibiotic prescribing. Also, distributing short, guideline-based recommendations. (Improving appropriate use and decreasing costs.)
- Restricting antibiotic use and using stronger infection control measures, which may be effective in reducing incidence of resistant infections in hospitals.
- Evaluating cost-effectiveness of antibiotic treatment alternatives, which must explicitly consider the costs of resistance.
- Undertaking further research to understand and alter incentives faced by patients and doctors in their use of antibiotics, including the barriers imposed by health plans on prescribing.
- Research to explore the potential effects of altering patent protection laws for antibiotics.

Conclusions

Antibiotics have long been the centrepiece of modern medicine and, with a concerted effort to apply AAT, can continue to be for many years. AAT is critical to ensure that every patient is treated with the right drug, and that resistance levels do not continue to rise dramatically. It is also crucial to keep the cost of medication at reasonable levels and to ensure equitable treatment of citizens across the socioeconomic spectrum on regional, national and international levels. The central pillars of AAT include achieving maximum therapeutic effect and minimal resistance through judicious selection of drugs and dosages, and ensuring optimal socioeconomic benefits through diligent surveillance, research and education programmes.

References

1. Craig WA. Pharmacokinetic/pharmacodynamic parameters: rationale for antibacterial dosing of mice and men. *Clin Infect Dis* 1998; **26**: 1–12.
2. Balter M, Hyland RH, Low DE, Renzi PM. Recommendations on the management of chronic bronchitis. A practical guide for Canadian physicians. *Can Med Assoc J* 1994; **15**[S10]: 1–23.
3. Anglim AN, Klym B, Byers KE *et al*. Effect of a vancomycin restrictions policy on ordering practices during an outbreak of vancomycin-resistant *Enterococcus faecium*. *Arch Intern Med* 1997; **157**: 1132–6.
4. Pestotnik SL, Classen DC, Evans RS, Burke JP. Implementing antibiotic practice guidelines through computer-assisted decision support: clinical and financial outcomes. *Ann Intern Med* 1996; **124**: 884–90.
5. Seppala H, Klaukka T, Vuopio-Varkila J *et al*. The effect of changes in the consumption of macrolide antibiotics on erythromycin resistance in group A streptococci in Finland. *N Engl J Med* 1997; **337**: 441–6.
6. Molstad S, Cars O. Major change in the use of antibiotics following a national programme: Swedish Strategic Programme for the Rational use of Antimicrobial Agents and Surveillance of Resistance (STRAMA). *Scand J Infect Dis* 1999; **31**: 191–5.

Minimizing the development of resistance with appropriate antibiotic use

DR STEPHEN H. ZINNER

HARVARD MEDICAL SCHOOL, MOUNT AUBURN HOSPITAL, 330 MOUNT AUBURN STREET, CAMBRIDGE, MA 02138, USA

When antibiotics were introduced into common medical practice more than 50 years ago, they were heralded as life-saving wonder drugs. Indeed, no-one can doubt the impact these drugs have had on longevity, medical advance and reduced morbidity and mortality associated with common infections of the respiratory and urinary tracts and the central nervous system. The clinical utility and general safety of antibiotics in the treatment of serious and other bacterial infections has led to the widespread incursion of these drugs into all aspects of medical practice. While their importance and life-preserving potential cannot be denied, the past 30 years have also seen dramatic increases in infections caused by antibiotic-resistant bacteria. The scourges of methicillin-resistant *Staphylococcus aureus* (MRSA), vancomycin-resistant enterococci (VRE), penicillin- and tetracycline-resistant gonococci, and multiply resistant gram-negative bacteria are well known and, recently, the widespread presence of penicillin-resistant pneumococci has taken centre stage. About 10 years ago it was impossible to imagine significant penicillin resistance in these organisms and, in fact, most laboratories did not even test for susceptibility during the preceding 40 years.

Inappropriate use of antibiotics

It is often difficult to quantify the role of inappropriate antibiotic use in the emergence of antibiotic-resistant bacteria. However, the selection pressure of high levels of exposure to these drugs is probably the factor leading to bacterial mutations responsible for many mechanisms of resistance. The frequently cited examples of excess vancomycin use and VRE[1], excess cephalosporin use and the emergence of SHV-1 extended spectrum β-lactamases[2,3], plus erythromycin use and resistant β-haemolytic streptococci[4], are well known. The relationship between optimal dose and duration of penicillin use in the treatment of pneumococcal infections might contribute to the emergence of penicillin resistance in these organisms[5]. In addition, the contribution of widespread antibiotic use in animal husbandry, vegetable and flower agriculture, cosmetics, over-the-counter first aid medications and even in battleship paint, as a barnacle retardant, cannot be underestimated[6,7].

There are very few controlled studies that prove definitively that 'appropriate' antibiotic use alone will reduce the presence or stem the emergence of antibiotic-resistant bacteria[8]. It is important that such studies be performed, and that realistic expectations are maintained for control measures that are introduced to reduce the problem of resistant bacteria.

Drug choice, dose and duration

The development of resistance is not necessarily related to the choice of a specific antibiotic or antibiotic class. It may be assumed that rapid-acting bactericidal agents are less likely to lead to the emergence of resistant strains compared with slower bacteriostatic agents, but it is clear that resistance has developed to third-generation cephalosporins and aminoglycosides as well as to tetracyclines and macrolides. Furthermore, whereas fluoroquinolones were originally thought to prevent plasmid-mediated resistance, in fact, resistance in staphylococci and pseudomonads does occur. Moreover, after more than 10 years of use, low-level resistance is being seen in *E. coli* and *S. pneumoniae*[9]. It is assumed that bacterial resistance is more likely to develop in the presence of subinhibitory concentrations or large inocula, or after long-term administration. However, it has not been proven that the use of high-dose, short course, rapidly bactericidal antibiotic therapy will prevent bacterial resistance from developing.

The importance of pharmacokinetics and pharmacodynamics in determining the antimicrobial effect has been stressed recently[10], and a few studies have investigated the impact of 'optimizing' pharmacodynamics on the selection of antibiotic-resistant bacteria. One such study suggested that if the ratio of the area under the curve (AUC) to the minimum inhibitory concentration (MIC) of ciprofloxacin (AUC/MIC ratio) approaches 100, then the likelihood of culturing resistant organisms from antibiotic-treated patients is much less than if the AUC/MIC ratio is lower[11]. This implies that the use of an agent that provides rapid bactericidal activity to eliminate all of the pathogenic organisms promptly might also be associated with a reduction in resistant organisms. While it might be naive to suggest that this approach would have widespread benefit on antimicrobial resistance rates, it is likely to be worthy of study in laboratory and clinical models.

Drlica and colleagues have introduced a new concept – the mutant prevention concentration (MPC). MPC can be defined as the concentration of antibiotic which produces no colony recovery when more than 10^{10} organisms are applied to agar plates[12]. A 'mutant selection window' can be described for antibiotic pharmacokinetics to define the area in the concentration–time curve above the MIC and below the MPC in which resistant mutants could be selected[13]. If this mutant selection window could be closed — that is drug concentration kept above the MPC — then resistant mutants could be prevented[13]. Theoretically, if agents that either exceed the MPC or remain active against bacteria with first- or second-order mutations were used preferentially or perhaps exclusively, then the emergence of resistance might be prevented. If this were true and possible, then a reorientation of the standard approach to antibiotic therapy might be required. At present, however, more laboratory and clinical data are needed before this paradigm can be suggested. Nonetheless, for some infections it does make sense to use preferentially an antibiotic that is highly active against the infecting organisms, at the appropriate dose that prevents the emergence of resistant organisms and for the shortest time to produce a beneficial clinical effect. Further clinical studies to prove this point are needed.

Recommendations

Strategies to minimize or eliminate antibiotic-resistant bacteria are being introduced by several organizations including the national Centers for Disease Control and Prevention (CDC), the World Health Organization (WHO), the Infectious Diseases Society of America and many political groups. Some of these guidelines stress the use of older, cheaper drugs for routine use in respiratory infections, and some stress the importance of ensuring that a bacterial infection is present (or even identified, wherever possible). Using a population dynamics approach, Levin has suggested that it might be very difficult for community interventions to have a major impact on antibiotic resistance, but nosocomial efforts to reduce resistance are more likely to succeed[14].

Conclusions

Undoubtedly, unnecessary use of antibiotics must be curtailed. Every effort should be made to educate doctors and healthcare providers, patients, and pharmaceutical companies so that bacterial infections are treated with potent, effective antibiotics, and that non-bacterial or trivial self-limiting infections are not. Definitive new studies to investigate the role of optimizing diagnostic techniques, effective vaccines, infection control methods, pharmacodynamics, drug selection, and new target development in this respect are sorely needed.

References

1. Fridkin SK, Edwards JR, Pichette SC et al. Determinants of vancomycin use in adult intensive care units in 41 United States hospitals. *Clin Infect Dis* 1999; **28**: 1119–25.
2. Medeiros AA. Evolution and dissemination of β-lactamases accelerated by generations of β-lactam antibiotics. *Clin Infect Dis* 1997; **24**(suppl 1): S19–45.
3. Rasheed JK, Jay C, Metchock B et al. Evolution of extended-spectrum β-lactam resistance (SHV-8) in a strain of *Escherichia coli* during multiple episodes of bacteremia. *Antimicrob Agents Chemother* 1997; **41**: 647–53.
4. Seppala H, Klaukka T, Lehtonen R et al. Outpatient use of erythromycin: link to increased erythromycin resistance in group A streptococci. *Clin Infect Dis* 1995; **21**: 1378–85.
5. Guillemot D, Carbon C, Balkau B et al. Low dosage and long treatment duration of β-lactam: risk factors for carriage of penicillin-resistant *Streptococcus pneumoniae*. *JAMA* 1998; **279**: 365–470.
6. DuPont HL, Steele JH. Use of antimicrobial agents in animal feeds: implications for human health. *Rev Infect Dis* 1987; **9**: 447–60.
7. Raloff J. Drugged waters: does it matter that pharmaceuticals are turning up in water supplies? *Science News* March 21, 1998; **153**: 187.
8. Phillips I. Lessons from the past: a personal view. *Clin Infect Dis* 1998; **27**(suppl 1): S2–4.
9. Chen DK, McGeer A, de Azavedo JC, Low DE. Decreased susceptibility of *Streptococcus pneumoniae* to fluoroquinolones in Canada. Canadian Bacterial Surveillance Network. *New Engl J Med* 1999; **341**: 233–9.
10. Craig WA. Pharmacokinetic/pharmacodynamic parameters: rationale for antibacterial dosing of mice and men. *Clin Infect Dis* 1998; **26**: 1–12.
11. Thomas JK, Forrest A, Bhavnani SM et al. Pharmacodynamic evaluation of factors associated with the development of bacterial resistance in acutely ill patients during therapy. *Antimicrob Agents Chemother* 1998; **42**(3): 521–7.
12. Dong Y, Zhao X, Domagala J, Drlica K. Effect of fluoroquinolone concentration on selection of resistant mutants of *Mycobacterium bovis* BCG and *Staphylococcus aureus*. *Antimicrob Agents Chemother* 1999; **43**: 1756–8.
13. Zhao X, Drlica K. A general strategy for restricting the selection of antibiotic-resistant mutants derived from fluoroquinolone studies. *Clin Infect Dis* 2001, **32**: (In Press).
14. Levin BR. Minimizing potential resistance — population dynamics view. *Clin Infect Dis* 2001, **32**: (In Press).

Achieving maximum therapeutic effect through appropriate antibiotic selection and use

DR STEVEN NELSON

JOHN H SEABURY PROFESSOR OF MEDICINE, SCHOOL OF MEDICINE IN NEW ORLEANS, 1901 PERDIDO STREET, SUITE 3205, NEW ORLEANS, LA 70112-1393, USA

Introduction

Will the twenty-first century see the end of the antibiotic age? The rise in microbes that are able to resist old and newer antibiotics has suggested to some that the clinical utility of these drugs may be limited in the near future. However, the informed clinician can still find the right drug regimen to control bacterial infection in the appropriate patient. To be successful, a pathogen must find a susceptible host. The essential feature of most infections is the successful multiplication of a microbe within that host. Disease occurs when signs and symptoms result from infection and its associated tissue damage and altered physiology. In choosing the appropriate antimicrobial agent for therapy of a given infection, several key factors must be considered. Namely, the most likely identity of the infecting organism, the potential antimicrobial susceptibility of the infecting organism, and host factors that influence the response to therapy.

The Big Picture

Effective antibiotic use depends on an understanding of the overall clinical context of the patient's illness. To maximize the therapeutic effect of an antimicrobial drug, the physician must consider its history of effectiveness in the institution and community that the patient and the physician share. The susceptibility of a specific microbe to a particular drug will vary among institutions or communities. The clinician must consider not only the individual patient's antibiotic treatment but also the overall patterns of antibiotic use in that hospital and community[1].

In many cases, there may be variations in susceptibility patterns between hospitals and the community or within the hospitals themselves. The emergence of gram-negative bacilli that are resistant to gentamicin is a good example of this. Most of the aminoglycoside-resistant organisms are found in hospitals, whereas most isolates from non-hospitalized patients remain susceptible to gentamicin. Within a hospital, the liberal use of antimicrobials in intensive care units has been associated with the rise of pathogens that are able to withstand many individual drugs[2]. Resistant bacteria have been found to occur more frequently in ICU patients than in other inpatients or outpatients[3]. Genetic variability is essential in order for microbial evolution to occur. Antimicrobial agents exert strong selective pressures on bacterial population, favoring those organisms that are capable of resisting them. Bacterial resistance can occur through several different mechanisms. It may arise when a single bacterium spontaneously mutates into a resistant form, and the selective pressure of antibiotics against its less resistant siblings allows the resistant organism to thrive. Such mutations are believed to account for the resistance to streptomycin, quinolones and rifampin. For other types of resistance, a microbe must achieve several successive mutations, each minutely reducing its susceptibility to a particular drug[4].

Bacteria can also acquire genetic material for resistance mutations from other resistant bacteria, through a process called conjugation, or from viruses with bacterial DNA in a process called transduction. Transformation, the process of incorporating free DNA from the environment, can also allow bacteria to acquire resistance. This horizontal acquisition of resistance depends upon the existence of local pools of resistant organisms often in the normal flora. The lower resistance levels seen in infections acquired in the community vis-à-vis those acquired in hospitals may reflect the decreased likelihood of horizontally acquired resistance[1]. A similar effect may be at work in the varying resistance levels among geographic regions, although these may also reflect localized patterns of antimicrobial use and specific responses to antibiotics.

In one study of the prevalence of *Streptococcus pneumoniae* in Atlanta, one quarter of all patients had strains that were penicillin-resistant. 26% of the isolates studied were also resistant to trimethoprim-sulfamethoxazole. Penicillin resistant pneumococci were found more frequently among whites than among blacks and multiply resistant microbes were found more frequently among white children under six than among black children in that age group. The researchers suggested that the racial differentiation might reflect differing economic status or access to health care, rather than an ethnically differentiated response to antibiotics[5].

The association of liberal use of antibiotics and the increased likelihood of resistance has sometimes led to the restriction of antibiotic prescriptions on an institutional or even national basis. In Finland, a concerted effort to restrict the use of erythromycin for treatment of outpatient infections was able to achieve a reduction in the incidence of erythromycin resistance[6]. In one American hospital with an outbreak of vancomycin-resistant enterococcal infections, the rate of resistance was significantly lowered by the introduction of controls for vancomycin prescriptions along with improved isolation and hygiene practices.

Which Microbe?

Ideally, the exact strain of microbe that is the cause of infection should be identified before an antimicrobial is prescribed. Several methods for the rapid identification of pathogenic bacteria in clinical specimens are available. Different strains of a single species may respond differently to a particular antibiotic. That is why it is particularly useful to determine the antimicrobial susceptibility of the actual infecting organism. Moreover, many diseases are not caused by microbial infections[8]. Additionally the improper use of antibiotics may mask the disease's true symptoms and mislead the clinician. All antibiotics also carry the risk of adverse effects of varying severity[4].

However, in most cases it may be impossible to determine the exact nature of the infecting organisms despite extensive testing and the life-threatening nature of an infection may not allow the clinician the time necessary to conduct tests to establish the identity of the microbe to be treated. In that situation, the clinician must embark on an empiric or initial therapy directed against the most probable pathogens in that particular patient. In a severely ill patient, where the cost of failure is great, a potent broad-spectrum agent is the wisest choice. The use of 'bacteriologic statistics' may also be helpful. The term 'bacteriologic statistics' refers to the application of knowledge of the organisms most likely to cause infections in a given clinical setting. Because the empiric antibiotic may render microbial cultures sterile while still allowing active organisms to multiply in the patient, specimens must be collected from the patient prior to the initiation of empiric therapy in order to optimize the opportunity to identify the organism[1].

Assessment of which pathogens are most likely sources of disease will depend on the physician's use of the clinical signs and symptoms displayed by the patient, the site of the infection, the underlying status of the host, and the physician's understanding of bacteriologic statistics[1]. For example a person with normal host defense mechanisms who develops a urinary tract infection most likely has an infection due to *Escherichia coli* and antimicrobial therapy should be selected accordingly. Similarly, a patient with an acute bacterial exacerbation of chronic bronchitis almost certainly has an infection due to one of three major bacterial pathogens-*Haemophilus influenzae*, *Moraxella catarrhalis*, or *Streptococcus pneumoniae*.

Which Drug?

Once the identity of the infecting microorganism is established, the empiric antibiotic regimen can now become more focused. This should be a narrow-spectrum antibiotic with a low adverse-effect profile to which the microbe is susceptible. Microbial susceptibility to a given drug may be established by disk-diffusion or dilution tests. These tests can provide the minimum inhibitory concentration (MIC), the level at which the tested drug can stop the growth of the tested microbe. Each drug-microbe combination has its own MIC. For example, the penicillin-resistant form of *S. pneumoniae* has an MIC of 2 ug/L against amoxicillin, but its MIC against cefaclor is 64 ug/L[9].

While the MIC is established in the laboratory, the actual clinical effect of the drug must be observed in the patient. Different drugs are characterized by different patterns of bactericidal activity. Some drugs such as the aminoglycosides, fluoroquinolones, and metronidazole (when used against anaerobic bacteria) show a direct relation between the level of concentration and the rate and extent of bactericidal activity. The higher the concentration, the more microbes die and the more quickly they die. Efficacy for these drugs correlates with the ratio of the peak concentration of the drug divided by the MIC.

For other drugs such as the beta-lactam antibiotics, macrolides, clindamycin, and vancomycin, bactericidal activity depends on the length of exposure, provided a minimum concentration is maintained. For these drugs, the killing rate quickly reaches a maximum relative to the levels of drug concentration achieved, and efficacy correlates with the time in which the patient's concentration of the drug exceeds the MIC[9].

These distinctions have obvious consequences for the dosage regiments of the drug chosen. For the first drug type, the dosage and frequency of administration should be designed to achieve maximum concentrations consistent with patient tolerance and the avoidance of toxicity. For the second type, the goal should be to maintain lower concentrations (but still above MIC) for the maximum period of time. These different patterns of concentration can be measured using the area under the curve (AUC), a number derived from the curve that graphs the level of drug concentration in the body over time. A more clinically important measure of some drugs' efficacy may be the area under the inhibitory time curve (AUIC). This number is the ratio of the AUC over the MIC, and thus combines the drug concentration, microbe susceptibility, and time factors.

An inappropriate choice of antibiotic can lead to worsened illness, increased microbial resistance, and costly therapy failure resulting in extra visits to the physician, extra tests, and extra drugs. Bacteria can resist the attack of an antibiotic by preventing the drug from reaching its target, by altering the target or by inactivating the drug. Understanding the mechanism of resistance can also influence the choice and use of antibiotics, as certain drugs have been developed to "minimize" the likelihood of resistance developing.

Which Infection?

The site of the infection determines not only the choice of the agent, but also its dose and the route by which it should be administered. For antimicrobial therapy to be effective, an adequate dose of the drug must be delivered to the site of infection. While MICs and AUCs generally reflect the level of drug in the patient's serum, the drug must reach the site of the infection in sufficient concentration to combat the infecting microbes. While subinhibitory levels of drugs have been shown to enhance the body's own defenses and impair microbial morphology and adherence, the better course is to ensure that the MIC is achieved at the infection site. Several studies have shown a significant correlation between attained antibacterial activity in bronchial secretions and efficacy of treatment. Specifically, clinical response has been correlated with bronchial levels of antimicrobials that exceed the MIC of the presumed pathogen. For some drugs such as spiromycin, the tissue concentration levels can exceed the serum levels. Thus, these drugs are clinically effective, even though the MIC is not reached in the serum.[1]

Antibiotic penetration into bronchial secretions is accomplished primarily by passive diffusion, which is critically dependent on serum antibiotic concentrations. However, blood flow into areas of infected lung may be significantly reduced because of hypoxic pulmonary vasoconstriction. Furthermore, many antibiotics penetrate the bronchial mucosa at a level of only 20% to 30% of maximally achieved systemic levels when given either orally or parenterally. Known factors that affect the ability of an antibiotic to cross the blood-lung barrier include molecular weight, lipophilicity, and protein binding. Bronchial inflammation may also cause alterations in tissue barriers and changes in the permeability of antibiotics. Once within the lung, antibiotics may be adversely affected by local pH conditions or bound by proteins present within purulent secretions. Rapid clearance as a result of cough and mucociliary transport may also contribute to antibiotic failures.

Which Patient?

It is obviously important to determine the identity and antimicrobial susceptibility of the pathogen causing a specific infection. Furthermore, optimal therapy is not attainable unless a number of host factors that influence the efficacy and toxicity of an antimicrobial agent are considered. Host factors can be classified into two categories: those that influence exposure and those that influence infection and the occurrence and severity of disease. Factors that influence human exposure to an infectious agent depend on contact with sources of infection within the environment (animal exposure, food or water consumption, socioeconomic status, travel) or the promotion of person-to-person transmission (child daycare attendance, closed living quarters, familial exposure, sexual activity). For most infections, two host factors play a key role in determining the likelihood of a clinical illness and the severity of that illness: the immune status of the host and the age at the time of infection. Typically, the highest levels of pathogenicity and virulence associated with the pathogen-host relationship tends to occur at the extremes of life-either very early when immune defense mechanisms are immature and not fully developed or at an older age, when they are deteriorating and undermined by the presence of significant co-morbidities.

Young and old patients also have different pharmacokinetics than the majority of patients. Elderly patients and children may have decreased levels of gastric acidity and weaker renal function. The gastric changes may enhance their absorption of such drugs as penicillin G or beta-lactam antibiotics administered orally, resulting in higher serum concentration levels. However, weak acid drugs such as ketoconazole are better absorbed at low pH levels and may be less well suited to these groups. Renal function also varies with age. Loss of renal function can allow renally cleared drugs such as the penicillins or cephalosporins to accumulate in the elderly patient. High serum levels may result in neurotoxic reactions. A similar risk is seen in newborns whose renal function has not yet reached mature status. Neonates also have underdeveloped hepatic function. Drugs that are handled by the liver may accumulate in the body and become toxic. For example, chloramphenicol, which is inactivated in the liver, may cause shock, cardiovascular collapse, or death in infants. Hepatic and renal impairment unrelated to age may also result in toxic levels of drug concentration[1]. Pregnant patients and nursing mothers also require special consideration when prescribing. All antibiotics cross the placenta and virtually all can appear in breast milk. Thus, the effect on the fetus or baby must also be a factor when choosing a drug for the mother. For example, tetracycline is known to cause renal damage, pancreatitis, and liver necrosis in some pregnant women. It also is known to affect the fetal or child's dentition.

The profiling of patients can be particularly useful for the determination of appropriate antibiotic therapy. For example, in the management of chronic bronchitis, Balter and colleagues identified risk factors such as poor pulmonary function, advanced age and comorbid medical illnesses, in stratifying patients and identifying appropriate therapy for each group of patients.[10] In one study, antibiotics were less effective in treating patients with acutely exacerbated chronic obstructive pulmonary disease if the patients also had a history of previous pneumonia or the use of home oxygen or maintenance steroids.[11] Similarly in 1993, the American Lung Association developed four subgroups of patients with community-acquired pneumonia based on age, need for hospitalization, severity of illness, and the presence of coexisting diseases. Antibiotic recommendations were made according to which subgroup the patient was in. In 1998, the Infectious Disease Society of America developed similar guidelines with the major criteria for antibiotic selection based on the severity of illness, curability, exposure, and the epidemiological setting.

Real-World Effectiveness

It is imperative that the clinician bear in mind all of the considerations discussed here when using antibiotics. An understanding of the clinical setting in which a patient receives treatment, the determination of the exact pathogen to be eradicated and its history of resistance, the site of infection, and the patient's individual ability to respond to therapy will all influence the course of treatment. Therapeutic effectiveness can be maximized by choosing and implementing the right drug regimen for the right patient in the right context.

References

1. Moellering RC Jr, Principles of Anti-Infective Therapy. In: Mandell GL, Bennett JE and Dolin R, eds. *Mandell, Douglas and Bennett's Principles and Practice of Infectious Diseases.* Philadelphia: McGraw-Hill, 1999: 200.
2. Gold HS and Moellering RC Jr. Antimicrobial-Drug Resistance. *NEJM* 1996; **335**(19): 1445-1453.
3. Archibald L, Phillips L, Monnet D *et al.* Antimicrobial Resistance in Isolates from Inpatients and Outpatients in the United States: Increasing Importance of the Intensive Care Unit. *Clin Infect Dis* 1997; **24**(2): 211-215.
4. Antimicrobial Agents: General Considerations. In: Hardman JG and Limbird LE, eds. *Goodman & Gilman's the Pharmacological Basis of Therapeutics* (9th Edn.). New York: Williams-Wilkens, 1999: 1032.
5. Hofmann J, Cetron MS, Farley MM *et al.* The Prevalence of Drug-Resistant *Streptococcus pneumoniae* in Atlanta. *NEJM* 1995; **333**(8): 481-486.
6. Seppala H, Klaukka T, Lehtonen R, *et al.* Outpatient Use of Erythromycin: Link to Increased Erythromycin Resistant Group A Streptococci. *Clin Infect Dis* 1995: **21**: 1378.
7. Anglim AM, Klym B, Byers KE *et al.* Effect of a Vancomycin Restrictions Policy on Ordering Practices During an Outbreak of Vancomycin-Resistant Enterococcus faecium. *Arch Intern Med* 1997; **157**: 1132-36.
8. Schentag JJ, Tillotson GS. Antibiotic Selection and Dosing for the Treatment of Acute Exacerbations of COPD. *Chest* 1997; **112**: 314S-9S.
9. Craig, WA. Pharmacokinetic/Pharmacodynamic Parameters: Rationale for the Antibacterial Dosing of Mice and Men. *Clin Infect Dis* 1998; **26**: 1-12.
10. Balter M, *et al.* Recommendations on the Management of Chronic Bronchitis. A Practical Guide for Canadian Physicians. *CMAJ* 1994; **15**[S10]: 1-23.
11. Dewan NA, Rafique S, Kanwar B *et al.* Acute Exacerbation of COPD: Factors Associated with Poor Treatment Outcome. *Chest* 2000; **117**(3): 662-671.
12. Thomas JK, Forrest A, Bhavnani SM *et al.* Pharmacodynamic Evaluation of Factors Associated with the Development of Bacterial Resistance in Acutely Ill Patients During Therapy. *Antimicrob Agents Chemother* 1998; **42**(3): 521-527.

Select the most appropriate antibiotic first

DR G. DOUGLAS CAMPBELL

PROFESSOR, LSU MEDICAL CENTER, 1501 KINGS HIGHWAY, ROOM 6341, SHREVEPORT, LA 71103, USA

Infectious diseases remain a major cause of morbidity and mortality despite significant improvements in healthcare. It is appreciated that the rapid institution of appropriate antimicrobial therapy can improve outcomes. The goal of such an approach is to cure the infection without incident and not promote resistance with the realization that a successful outcome depends not just upon the antimicrobial agent alone, but also upon host (adequacy of host defences) and bacterial related (antibiotic resistance) factors as well. Unfortunately, the approach taken to determine the choice of antimicrobial agent(s) remains controversial.

Appropriate antibiotic selection

Ideally, the most appropriate antimicrobial agent would be a narrow spectrum drug, selected once the offending pathogen was identified and any antimicrobial resistance was known. The rational of directed therapy includes a reduction in polypharmacy, a lower incidence of adverse drug reactions, less antibiotic selection pressure and reduced costs. In an ideal world, such an approach would be the preferred method for treating infectious illness.

In the real world, however, this approach is just not possible for many types of infectious disease. A good example of this concerns the treatment of community-acquired pneumonia, which can be caused by a broad spectrum of potentially infectious agents. The limitations for using directed therapy are numerous. Identification of the offending pathogen, and certainly knowledge of its antimicrobial resistance, is usually unavailable at the time antimicrobial choices are made. If serological studies are performed, the results are not available for weeks, long after the patient has either recovered or succumbed to their infection. No single test can identify all potential infectious agents. Extensive testing is expensive and many common tests lack sensitivity and/or specificity. In addition, these tests may determine an aetiology only

50% of the time. In some patient populations, more than one-third of all pneumonia is caused by at least two very different pathogens. Thus, most antimicrobial choices by necessity are empirical and broad spectrum.

If there are limitations with directed therapy, is empirical therapy inappropriate? At the dawn of the antibiotic era, most agents had a limited spectrum and the efficacy of an antibiotic was determined by knowing its spectrum of activity and then determining susceptibility endpoints such as the mean inhibitory concentration (MIC) and mean bacteriocidal concentration (MBC) of the organism. These are measurements of an antibiotic's pharmocodynamics, ie the study of the biochemical and physiological effects of drugs and their mechanisms of action (site of action, MIC, antibiotic breakpoints, bacteriocidal vs. bacteriostatic). If the MIC of an organism was less than a predetermined breakpoint, which was based upon the peak serum level for that antibiotic, then the organism was considered susceptible and the doctor would initiate therapy. Use of susceptibility endpoints was simple to understand and allowed for the monitoring of antibiotic resistance, but these same end-points were only part of the picture.

Advances in therapy

With the introduction of aminoglycosides and the recognition of ototoxicity and renal toxicity from high aminoglycoside levels, peak and trough measurements became common. Ultimately studies showed that improved efficacy was dependent upon the peak aminoglycoside level and the fact that lower incidence of drug-related side effects correlated with trough levels. From these investigations, it became common practice to dose aminoglycosides based upon the drug's pharmacokinetics using the patient's age, gender, weight and serum creatinine[1].

The past two decades have witnessed an increase in understanding of antibiotic pharmacokinetics: the action of a drug in the body over a period of time including the process of absorption, distribution, localization in tissues, biotransformation and excretion. One of the first findings addressed bacteriocidal activity[2]. It was noted that with some classes of antimicrobial agents, the higher the drug concentration was above the MIC, the greater the extent and rate of killing. Other classes of agents showed minimal differences in the rate and extent of killing with increasing drug concentrations but demonstrated that the duration of time spent above the MIC affected the killing rate: this mechanism was termed time-dependent killing. This information had direct clinical relevance, because it allowed once-daily dosing of aminoglycosides, which has now become common practice. Studies of pharmacokinetics have now been extended to all classes of antimicrobial agents.

A second finding was the persistent activity that some antibiotic agents had against pathogens hours after therapy was discontinued. Post-antibiotic effect (PAE), as it was called, was first described with penicillin effects on *Streptococcus pneumoniae* and staphylococci[3]. Essentially all antibiotics exert a PAE on common gram-positive cocci, but only agents that inhibit protein or nucleic acid synthesis have a prolonged PAE for gram-negative organisms. These include the following classes: aminoglycosides, fluoroquinolones, tetracyclines, macrolides, chloramphenicol, rifampicin and the carbapenems. Most studies of PAE have been performed either in vitro or using animal models of infection. In addition to PAE, some agents have been shown to slow bacterial growth and produce morphological changes at sub-MIC levels, which can further prolong the PAE (known as the post-antibiotic sub MIC effect, PAE-SME)[4]. Finally some classes of agents can cause bacteria to be more susceptible to phagocytosis or intracellular leucocyte attack in the post-treatment period. This phenomenon is called the post-antibiotic leucocyte effect (PALE)[5].

Taken together, these pharmacokinetic findings have affected dosing of certain antibiotics. For example, infrequent dosing at high concentration should be effective for an antimicrobial with concentration-dependent killing antibiotics and a good PAE (aminoglycosides and fluoroquinolones). This has led to single dose daily therapy with aminoglycosides. With the fluoroquinolones, use of either the ratio of the peak serum concentration to the MIC of the pathogen (C_{max}/MIC) or the area under the curve (AUC) above the MIC for 24 hours to the MIC ratio (AUIC), has been suggested as a method for determining effective therapy[6-8]. For agents whose killing is time-dependent (above the MIC) and who exhibit little PAE for gram-negative bacilli, frequent dosing with lower concentrations is preferable – for example, β-lactams should be given regularly at low doses.

The role of resistance

In addition to the advances made in pharmacokinetic measurements and the rapid rise in antimicrobial resistance, a better understanding has developed of both the pressures that promote resistance and the evolution of the mechanisms of resistance. It is appreciated that in the population of bacteria causing an infection, there is a range of natural resistance. Low dosing or prolonged periods of time at sub-MIC levels, especially for agents without a PAE, are associated with an increased risk for the development of resistance. Inappropriate empirical therapy, which is frequently reported in children with otitis infections or in adults with the 'flu', can also promote resistance in the resident flora. These resistance mechanisms can be transferred to pathogenic organisms in a variety of ways. This has led to national efforts to limit and change antimicrobial therapy in clinical settings. This risk is especially common in crowded settings (such as prisons) or settings where there is close contact (such as day care centres).

Conclusions

Is empirical therapy inappropriate? Until more rapid and sensitive diagnostic tests become available, doctors will have to rely on empirical therapy for the treatment of certain infectious diseases. The antibiotics available today have a broader spectrum of activity than previous agents and the understanding of pharmacokinetic and pharmacodynamic issues place doctors in a better position to select 'appropriate' treatments. In addition, a number of medical societies concerned about this problem have developed guidelines for treating a variety of infectious diseases. A major problem today is the increasing incidence of resistance that is driven by inappropriate empirical or prophylactic usage where infection is probably not present and the role of appropriate antimicrobial therapy has been questioned. The current conditions under which antibiotics are used require careful evaluation of a host of circumstances before agent administration. Appropriate selection of antibiotics should be based on available knowledge of both the patient and the offending pathogen(s), bearing in mind local resistance patterns and known interactions.

References

1. Smith CR, Lipsky JJ, Lietman PS. Relationship between aminoglycoside-induced nephrotoxicity and auditory toxicity. *Antimicrob Agents Chemother* 1979; **15**: 780–2.
2. Craig WA, Gudmundsson S. Postantibiotic effect. In: Lorian V, ed. *Antibiotics in laboratory medicine*. 4th ed. Baltimore: Williams and Wilkins, 1996: 296–329.
3. Mcdonald PJ, Craig WA, Kunin CM. Persistent effect of antibiotics on *Staphylococcus aureus* after exposure for limited periods of time. *J Infect Dis* 1977; **135**: 217–23.
4. Odenholt-Tornqvist I, Lowdin E, Cars O. Postantibiotic sub-MIC effects of vancomycin, roxithromycin, sparfloxacin, and amikacin. *Antimicrob Agents Chemother* 1992; **36**: 1852–8.
5. McDonald PJ, Wetherall BL, Pruul H. Postantibiotic leukocyte enhancement: increased susceptibility of bacteria pretreated with antibiotics to activity of leukocytes. *Rev Infect Dis* 1981; **3**: 38–44.
6. Hyatt JM, McKinnon PS, Zimmer GS *et al*. The importance of pharmacokinetic/pharmacodynamic surrogate markers to outcome: focus on antibacterial agents. *Clin Pharmacokinet* 1995; **28**: 143–60.
7. Drusano GL, Johnson DE, Rosen M, Standiford HC. Pharmacodynamics of a fluoroquinolone antimicrobial agent in a neutropenic rat model of Pseudomonas sepsis. *Antimicrob Agents Chemother* 1993; **37**: 483–90.
8. Firsov AA, Vostrov SN, Shevchenko AA *et al*. A new approach to in vitro comparisons of antibiotics in dynamic models: equivalent area under the curve/MIC breakpoints and equiefficient doses of trovafloxacin and ciprofloxacin against bacteria of similar susceptibilities. *Antimicrob Agents Chemother* 1998; **42**: 2841–7.

Criteria for appropriate antibiotic use in hospital and managed-care settings

DR ANTONIO ANZUETO

ASSOCIATE PROFESSOR OF MEDICINE, UNIVERSITY OF TEXAS — HSC AT SAN ANTONIO,
7400 MERTON MINTER BLVD, SAN ANTONIO, TX 78284, USA

For the past half-century, doctors have observed with concern the proliferation of microbes able to resist antibiotic therapy. In the World Health Organization's Global Burden of Disease Study of worldwide future mortality and disability, infectious diseases constituted five of the top 10 causes of years lost due to disease or injury. The reality of drug resistance spreading to tuberculosis, malaria, or pneumococcal infection is leading to even higher losses[1]. While resistant pathogens now create a serious problem for the whole community, these micro-organisms pose a particular danger for those in healthcare facilities. Unless stringent precautions are taken in patient care and drug prescribing, hospital environments increase the likelihood of pathogens acquiring resistance and provide a ready means for inter-host transmission of resistant pathogens.

Are hospitals hotbeds of resistance?

A rising number of studies are showing that resistant bacteria are occurring primarily in the most vulnerable hospital patients – one US study of patients at eight hospitals found that isolates from intensive care unit (ICU) patients were the most likely to show resistant micro-organisms. Resistant microbes were seen less frequently in non-ICU inpatient isolates, and outpatient isolates showed the smallest incidence of resistant colonization or infection. For example, methicillin-resistant *Staphylococcus aureus* (MRSA) was observed in 33% of inpatient isolates but in only 14.5% of outpatient isolates[3].

Hospitals and other institutional settings represent a focus for the effects of selective pressure, one of the factors that contribute to the emergence of resistant microbes. Selective pressure is the mechanism by which antibiotics kill less resistant competitors of a newly mutated resistant strain of pathogen. In the absence of the drug's bacteriocidal effect, the new strain would be forced to compete with a much larger population of microbes. However, due to the antibiotic's elimination of their more susceptible 'siblings', the resistant bacteria are able to flourish[4]. The use of empirical antibiotic therapy and broad-spectrum antimicrobial agents in hospitals may increase the effect of selective pressure. Doctors continue to prescribe excessive or inappropriate drugs, despite the establishment of guidelines, the implementation of restricted prescribing procedures and efforts to educate the profession. Usually, the prescribing doctor's immediate concern is the individual patient rather than the balance between that patient's needs and the effects of microbial resistance for the whole patient population[2].

In addition to greater mortality rates, antibiotic-resistant bacterial infections are associated with prolonged hospitalization and increased healthcare costs relative to antibiotic-sensitive infections. Recently, the authors of a US study estimated that the emergence of antibiotic resistance among *Pseudomonas aeruginosa* increased hospital charges by $11,981 per patient[5]. Other authors have also reported increased medical care costs associated with antibiotic-resistant infections, including oxacillin-resistant *Staphylococcus aureus*[6]. Currently, the annual cost for control and treatment of infections caused by antibiotic-resistant bacteria in the US is estimated to be between $100m and $30bn[7]. The increased cost of infections caused by antibiotic-resistant bacteria has been attributed primarily to prolonged hospitalization and greater antibiotic costs. Ibrahim *et al* evaluated the relationship between adequate antimicrobial treatment for bloodstream infections and clinical outcomes among patients requiring ICU admission[8]. The investigators found that 29.9% of patients received inadequate antimicrobial treatment for their bloodstream infection. These patients had a mortality of 61.9%, vs. 28.4% for the patients who received adequate therapy (relative risk 2.18; 95% CI 1.77–2.69; $p<0.001$), and furthermore, prolonged hospital stays. The report by Goldmann *et al*[2] concluded that basic infection control remains inadequate and allows the person-to-person transfer of pathogens. Staff frequently fail to wash their hands before and after patient contact, do not use gloves, and neglect to exercise adequate precautions in overcrowded wards or with incontinent or mechanically ventilated patients. One particularly acute source of risk is the patient who is colonized but not clinically infected with a resistant organism. The absence of overt symptoms reduces the likelihood that staff will exercise appropriate precautions[2].

Overcoming resistance

Rapid identification of microorganisms is one method of limiting the use of empirical antibiotic therapy. As soon as a pathogen has been isolated, the treating doctor can switch from empirical to therapeutic prescribing. A study of 14,069 elderly pneumonia patients found that those whose blood cultures were collected within 24 hours of attending hospital were 10% less likely to die within 30 days, than patients whose cultures were taken 24 hours or later. A 15% reduction in mortality was also associated with the prescription of antibiotics within eight hours of arrival. The authors concluded that microbiological monitoring using blood cultures can be used to guide empirical antibiotic therapy in cases of resistant microbes[9].

A sophisticated computerized system of managing antimicrobial use was instituted at a teaching hospital in Utah, US[11]. The programmes used rules, algorithms and predictive models and allowed doctors to input patient-specific clinical information. The programmes also tracked relevant patient variables such as renal status and adverse events, and flagged excessive or suboptimal doses. Over the seven years from 1988 to 1994, during which 63,759 patients (39.3%) received antibiotics, antibiotic use improved by several measures. While initially doctors ignored 70% of the system's alerts, by 1994 only 1 in 1,000 alerts would not result in a change of prescription. The average duration of antibiotic use after surgery, the incidence of antibiotic-associated adverse drug events, and mortality all fell significantly. The defined daily drug dose per 100 occupied bed days declined from 35.9 in 1988 to 27.7 in 1994. The antibiotic costs per treated patient (adjusted for inflation) were successfully cut from $122.66 in 1988 to $51.90 in 1994.

Formulary issues

The average hospital spends up to a fifth of its budget on drugs, and antibiotics account for up to half of this expense[11]. Financial pressures may lead to a reduction in the number of antibiotics available for prescription, but such limitation of drug choice may lead to inadequate or failed therapy with costly consequences such as longer lengths of stay[10]. Failed antibiotic therapy has also been linked to the promotion of resistance. In one study of 107 acutely ill patients, 32 of 128 initially susceptible microbes isolated acquired resistance to each antibiotic used against them[12]. However, isolates from patients who received several separate antibiotics simultaneously were significantly less likely to acquire resistance. The authors hypothesized that polytherapy was more effective at forestalling resistance because at least one of the drugs administered was likely to achieve a concentration sufficient to overcome the effect of selective pressure.

Conclusion

Appropriate antibiotic use — in the form of controlled measures such as the imposition of systematic barriers to improper prescribing — has been shown to be possible in hospitals and managed-care settings. Such measures are particularly important in these settings, which have traditionally been the foci for resistance development. Concerted efforts across regions, nations and around the world will ensure that antibiotic use will continue to be a valuable facet of modern healthcare in all locations for generations to come.

References

1. Murray CJL, Lopez AD. Alternative projections of mortality and disability by cause 1990–2020: Global Burden of Disease Study. *Lancet* 1997; **349**: 1498–1504.
2. Goldmann DA, Weinstein RA, Wenzel RP *et al.* Strategies to prevent and control the emergence and spread of antimicrobial-resistant microorganisms in hospitals: a challenge to hospital leadership. *JAMA* 1996; **275(3)**: 234–40.
3. Archibald L, Phillips L, Monnet D *et al.* Antimicrobial resistance in isolates from inpatients and outpatients in the United States: increasing importance of the intensive care unit. *Clin Infect Dis* 1997; **24(2)**: 211–5.
4. Tenover FC, Hughes JM. The challenges of emerging infectious diseases: development and spread of multiply-resistant pathogens. *JAMA* 1996; **275(4)**: 300–4.
5. Carmeli Y, Troillet N, Karchmer AW *et al.* Health and economic outcomes of antibiotic resistance in *Pseudomonas aeruginosa*. *Arch Intern Med* 1999; **159**: 1127–32.
6. Holemberg SD, Solomon SL, Blake PA. Health and economic impact of antimicrobial resistance. *Rev Infect Dis* 1987; **9**: 1065–78.
7. Publication OTA-H 629. *Impact of antibiotic-resistant bacteria: thanks to penicillin, he will come again!* Washington, DC: Office of Technology Assessment, Congress, 1995.
8. Ibrahim E, Sherman G *et al.* The influence of inadequate antimicrobial treatment of bloodstream infections on patient outcomes in the ICU setting. *Chest* 2000; **118**: 146–55. *[Dr Anzueto – Please supply 3rd author name]*
9. Meehan TP, Fine MJ, Krumholz HM *et al.* Quality of care, process, and outcomes in elderly patients with pneumonia. *JAMA* 1997; **278**: 2080–4.
10. Anglim AN, Klym B, Byers KE *et al.* Effect of a vancomycin restrictions policy on ordering practices during an outbreak of vancomycin-resistant *Enterococcus faecium*. *JAMA* 1997; **157(10)**: 1132–6.
11. Pestotnik SL, Classen DC, Evans RS *et al.* Implementing antibiotic practice guidelines through computer-assisted decision support: clinical and financial outcomes. *Ann Intern Med* 1996; **124(10)**: 884–90.
12. Thomas JK, Forrest A, Bhavnani SM *et al.* Pharmacodynamic evaluation of factors associated with the development of bacterial resistance in acutely ill patients during therapy. *Antimicrob Agents Chemother* 1998; **42(3)**: 521–7.

Reducing the economic burden through appropriate antibiotic use

DR JOSEPH A. PALADINO

DIRECTOR OF CLINICAL OUTCOMES AND PHARMACOECONOMICS, STATE UNIVERSITY OF NEW YORK AT BUFFALO, CPL ASSOCIATES LLC, 3980 SHERIDAN DRIVE, AMHERST, NY 14226, USA

In order for antibiotic use to be considered 'appropriate' a number of conditions must be met (Table 1). There are numerous clinical, social and economic benefits to be realized from rapid-acting, optimally effective, yet safe, antimicrobial regimens. Infections caused by resistant bacteria are associated with increased morbidity, mortality and healthcare expenditures.

Table 1 Initial conditions for appropriate antibiotic usage

- Antibiotic treatment is genuinely needed.
- The specific antibiotic chosen:
  ✓ has activity against the known/suspected pathogen
  ✓ will attain therapeutic concentrations at the site of infection
  ✓ has documented clinical efficacy for the intended use.
- The patient:
  ✓ does not have a history of adverse reaction to the compound or its cousins
  ✓ is able to have the agent administered (ie intravenous access or functioning enteral tract available).

Prompt initiation and appropriate treatment is required

In an early observation of aminoglycoside therapy, Noone *et al* determined that adequate therapy required achieving peak concentrations of ≥5 mg/ml within 72 hours of initiating gentamicin for the treatment of septicaemia, urinary tract infection (UTI) or wound infections, and that a peak concentration of ≥8 mg/ml should be attained for the treatment of pneumonia. Patients for whom these goals were reached had an 84% cure rate, compared to 23% cure in those who had not received adequate therapy[1].

More recent studies have examined whether or not prompt or delayed initiation of antibiotic therapy has an effect on clinical outcome. Administering antibiotics within 8 hours of admission to a hospital was associated with improved survival of elderly patients with pneumonia[2]. A review by Kollef indicated that patients with ventilator-associated pneumonia who had inadequate initial antimicrobial therapy were associated with a higher mortality rate (24.7%) than those who received adequate therapy (16.2%, $p=0.039$)[3].

Integration of pharmacodynamics and pharmacokinetics

Clinical application of pharmacological principles can produce further improvements in outcome. A key pharmacokinetic parameter, area under the curve (AUC), provides a measurement of the amount of drug available systemically in the patient. A key pharmacodynamic parameter, minimum inhibitory concentration (MIC), provides a measurement of the drug's in vitro potency. Integration of these two parameters can provide a measurement of the in vivo potency of an antimicrobial agent.

Antimicrobials exhibit either concentration- or time-dependent activity, and may have post-antibiotic effects towards specific micro-organisms[4]. AUC (pharmacokinetics) and MIC (pharmacodynamics) can be integrated by a ratio of AUC_{24} to MIC, also known as the area under the inhibitory curve (AUIC)[5]. Regardless of the type of activity, AUIC has been shown to be an accurate predictor of bacteriological and clinical response[4-11]. The first prospective study of AUIC was undertaken in patients hospitalized with pneumonia and treated with cefmenoxime (an investigational cephalosporin). Clinical response, as represented by reduced length of hospital stay, was improved with AUIC compared to standard dosing[6]. Economic analysis of this data demonstrated AUIC dosing to be cost-effective, with a net per patient saving in excess of $2,100 (corrected for the year 2000)[12].

Many investigators are performing AUIC studies with the goal of finding the breakpoint which predicts a successful outcome, usually measured by bacteriological eradication. However, for optimal therapy, the goals should be accompanied by speed of bacterial kill (Table 2) and, subsequently, a more rapid clinical response. These typically require somewhat higher AUIC values than those for minimum efficacy. In a study of hospitalized patients with predominately gram-negative pneumonia, AUIC values for ciprofloxacin of >250 were associated with a more rapid bacteriological eradication rate and patient response than lower values[7]. Economic assessment of these patients revealed net savings far in excess of the savings associated with cefmenoxime[13]. An explanation for the difference may be found in an analysis comparing the speed of kill of the two agents. At identical AUIC values (>250), ciprofloxacin was associated with a much more rapid eradication of

Table 2 Benefits of rapid eradication of infection

Beneficiary	Benefits
Patient	Reduced morbidity
	Reduced mortality
	Improved quality of life
Healthcare system	Fewer inpatient treatment days
	Fewer outpatient treatment days
	Lower direct medical costs
	Less frequent antimicrobial resistance
Society	Quicker return of individual to productivity

bacteria than cefmenoxime[14]. In a separate study of patients with acute bacterial exacerbations of chronic bronchitis, including many gram-positive bacteria, the AUIC of grepafloxacin required for rapid bacterial eradication (175) was higher than that for minimal acceptable cure (75)[9].

Drug potency and resistance

Given that bacterial eradication is enhanced by high AUIC values, and that non-viable bacteria cannot develop resistance, it can be inferred that higher AUIC values are associated with a decrease in resistance. This association was demonstrated in a recent study[15] and its value in preventing the development of antimicrobial resistance has been embraced[16].

Multicentre studies have examined the hospital-wide impact of using fluoroquinolone agents of various potencies. As measured by AUIC, ciprofloxacin is approximately four-fold more potent than ofloxacin against *Pseudomonas aeruginosa*. A benchmarking study of 109 US hospitals evaluated the impact of formulary conversion from ciprofloxacin to ofloxacin[17]. Hospitals made the change in order to take advantage of the lower price of ofloxacin, but lower prices do not necessarily ensure lower costs[18]. Expenditure for fluoroquinolones, non-fluoroquinolone anti-*Pseudomonal* antibiotics and total antibiotics either remained the same or, in some cases, actually increased as ofloxacin use increased[17]. Moreover, ofloxacin use was associated significantly with increased resistance of *Pseudomonas aeruginosa*[17].

A subsequent study of 156 US hospitals found a significantly greater association between increased expenditure on levofloxacin or ofloxacin and increased resistance of *Pseudomonas aeruginosa*, a result not replicated with ciprofloxacin, which is a more potent anti-*Pseudomonal* agent[19].

Do new agents offer superior efficacy?

Several recent studies demonstrate the superiority of new fluoroquinolones (such as levofloxacin) over established antimicrobials (such as cephalosporins and macrolides). A large study of inpatients and outpatients with community-acquired pneumonia, compared iv/po levofloxacin with iv ceftriaxone and/or po cefuroxime axetil (with or without erythromycin or doxycycline). Levofloxacin exhibited a significantly greater clinical success rate[20]. In a another study of inpatients with community-acquired pneumonia, clinical success rates similar to those of the previous study were observed[21], and a separate economic analysis found gatifloxacin to be significantly more cost-effective than ceftriaxone/macrolide[22]. Fluoroquinolone monotherapy may also be associated with decreased mortality and fewer hospitalizations, according to a meta-analysis of four multinational community-acquired pneumonia trials in which patients received either moxifloxacin or a comparator agent (amoxicillin or clarithromycin). The mortality and hospitalization rates were 0.57% and 0.86% for the moxifloxacin-treated patients compared to 1.7% ($p=0.045$) and 1.7% ($p=0.02$) for the comparator-treated patients[23].

Conclusion

With the clinical goal in mind, appropriate antimicrobial therapy should result in complete eradication of the infecting pathogen as rapidly as patient safety will allow. The faster the patient recovers from infection and returns to being a productive member of society, the fewer healthcare resources they will require. Furthermore, eradicated bacteria are 'dead' and unable to develop or spread resistance. In addition to providing effective therapy, numerous benefits will result from antimicrobial regimens that eradicate infectious pathogens (Table 2). Antimicrobial management programmes should not allow concern for drug prices to take precedence over this goal.

References

1. Noone P, Parsons TMC, Pattison JR et al. Experience in monitoring gentamicin therapy during treatment of serious gram-negative sepsis. *BMJ* 1974; **1**: 477-81.
2. Meehan TP, Fine MJ, Krumholz HM et al. Quality of care, process, and outcomes in elderly patients with pneumonia. *JAMA* 1997; **278**: 2080-4.
3. Kollef MH, Ward S. Antibiotic changes based on the findings of mini-bronchial alveolar lavage cultures are associated with increased patient mortality. *CHEST* 1998; **113**: 412-20.
4. Craig WA. Pharmacokinetic/pharmacodynamic parameters: rationale for antibacterial dosing of mice and men. *Clin Infect Dis* 1998; **26**: 1-12.
5. Schentag JJ, Nix DE, Adelman MH. Mathematical examination of dual individualization principles (I): relationships between AUC above MIC and area under the inhibitory curve for cefmenoxime, ciprofloxacin, and tobramycin. *DICP* 1991; **25**: 1050-7.
6. Schentag JJ, Smith IL, Swanson DJ et al. Role for dual individualization with cefmenoxime. *Am J Med* 1984; **77**(suppl 6A): 43-50.

7. Forrest A, Nix DE, Ballow CH et al. Pharmacodynamics of intravenous ciprofloxacin in seriously ill patients. *Antimicrob Agents Chemother* 1993; **37**: 1073-81.

8. Hyatt JM, McKinnon PS, Zimmer GS, Schentag JJ. The importance of pharmacokinetic/pharmacodynamic surrogate markers to outcome. Focus on antibacterial agents. *Clin Pharmacokinet* 1995; **28**: 143-60.

9. Forrest A, Chodosh S, Amantea MA et al. Pharmacokinetics and pharmacodynamics of oral grepafloxacin in patients with acute bacterial exacerbations of chronic bronchitis. *J Antimicrob Chemother* 1997; **40**(suppl A): 45-57.

10. Madras-Kelly KJ, Ostergaard BE, Baeker Hovde L, Rotschafer JC. Twenty-four-hour area under the concentration-time curve/MIC ratio as a generic predictor of fluoroquinolone antimicrobial effect by using three strains of *Pseudomonas aeruginosa* and an in vitro pharmacodynamic model. *Antimicrob Agents Chemother* 1996; **40**: 627-32.

11. Preston SL, Drusano GL, Berman AL et al. Pharmacodynamics of levofloxacin. *JAMA* 1998; **279**: 125-9.

12. Paladino JA, Fell RE. Pharmacoeconomic analysis of cefmenoxime dual individualization in the treatment of nosocomial pneumonia. *Ann Pharmacother* 1994; **28**: 384-9.

13. Paladino JA, Zimmer GS, Schentag JJ. The economic potential of dual individualization methodologies. *PharmacoEconomics* 1996; **6**: 539-45.

14. Goss TF, Forrest A, Nix DE et al. Mathematical examination of dual individualization principles (II): the rate of bacterial eradication at the same area under the inhibitory curve is more rapid for ciprofloxacin than for cefmenoxime. *Ann Pharmacother* 1994; **28**: 863-8.

15. Thomas JK, Forrest A, Bhavnani SM et al. Pharmacodynamic evaluation of factors associated with the development of bacterial resistance in acutely ill patients during therapy. *Antimicrob Agents Chemother* 1998; **42**: 521-7.

16. Burgess DS. Pharmacodynamic principles of antimicrobial therapy in the prevention of resistance. *Chest* 1999; **115**: 19-23S.

17. Rifenburg RP, Paladino JA, Bhavnani SM et al. Influence of fluoroquinolone purchasing patterns on antimicrobial expenditures and *Pseudomonas aeruginosa* susceptibility. *Am J Health Syst Pharm* 1999; **56**: 2217-23.

18. Dickson M, Redwood H. Pharmaceutical reference prices. How do they work in practice? *PharmacoEconomics* 1998; **14**: 471-9.

19. Bhavnani SM, Paladino JA, Forrest A et al. Association between fluoroquinolone expenditures and ciprofloxacin susceptibility of *Pseudomonas aeruginosa* among US hospitals. In: *Program and abstracts of the thirty-ninth interscience conference on antimicrobial agents and chemotherapy, San Francisco, CA, 1999.* Abstract 182. Washington, DC: American Society for Microbiology, 1999: 734.

20. File TM Jr, Segreti J, Dunbar L et al. A multicenter, randomized study comparing the efficacy and safety of intravenous and/or oral levofloxacin versus ceftriaxone and/or cefuroxime axetil in treatment of adults with community-acquired pneumonia. *Antimicrob Agents Chemother* 1997; **41**: 1965-72.

21. Fogarty C, Dowell ME, Ellison WT et al. Treating community-acquired pneumonia in hospitalized patients: gatifloxacin vs ceftriaxone/clarithromycin. *J Respir Dis* 1999; **20**(suppl): S60-9.

22. Dresser LD, Niederman MS, Paladino JA. Cost-effectiveness of gatifloxacin versus ceftriaxone with a macrolide for the treatment of community-acquired pneumonia. *Chest* 2001; **119**: 1439-48.

23. Niederman M, Church J, Kaufmann J et al. Does appropriate antibiotic treatment influence outcome in community-acquired pneumonia? *Respir Med* 2000; **94**(suppl): A14.

Socioeconomic issues related to antibiotic use

DR SHELBY D. REED

RESEARCH ASSOCIATE, PROGRAM IN PHARMACEUTICAL OUTCOMES RESEARCH AND POLICY, UNIVERSITY OF WASHINGTON, PO BOX 357630, SEATTLE, WA 98195-7630, USA

DR SEAN D. SULLIVAN

ASSOCIATE PROFESSOR, PROGRAM IN PHARMACEUTICAL OUTCOMES RESEARCH AND POLICY, UNIVERSITY OF WASHINGTON, PO BOX 357630, SEATTLE, WA 98195-7630, USA

DR RAMANAN LAXMINARAYAN

FELLOW, ENERGY AND NATURAL RESOURCES DIVISION, RESOURCES FOR THE FUTURE, 1616 P ST NW, WASHINGTON, DC 20036, USA

There are many varied and dynamic socioeconomic factors that foster the emergence and persistence of inappropriate antibiotic use. These range from political motivations, legal liability and resource constraints that impact upon decisions made at the level of government agencies, private industry, hospitals and managed-care organizations in developed countries to poor environmental and socioeconomic conditions in developing countries. In addition, organizational and medical policies may indirectly promote the injudicious use of antibiotics.

Although antibiotic resistance is widely considered to be a critical issue affecting public health worldwide, relatively little work has been undertaken to evaluate the costs associated with it. There is a role for surveillance to track resistance patterns and develop the data infrastructure with which to conduct relevant research.

Cost–benefit considerations

Appropriate antibiotic use carries both benefits and costs. Effective treatment benefits not just the patient, but society also, because of the potential of successful treatment (or prophylaxis)

to reduce transmission of the infection to other healthy individuals. On the cost side, antibiotic use increases selection pressure on bacteria thereby increasing their resistance to antibiotics[1]. These resistance-related costs are in addition to the cost of buying and administering the drug. Theoretically, optimal conditions would exist if cost–benefit trade-offs functioned to promote the judicious use of antibiotics, but economic factors usually operate to decrease appropriate use.

From a patient's perspective, the decision to request an antibiotic is based on the perceived benefit associated with each day of expedited recovery from infection and, in the US at least, the cost of treatment. Even so, in the US, insurance cover for prescription drugs shields the patient from direct responsibility for their cost, and further distorts patients' incentive to consider resistance. At the same time, doctors face few incentives to withhold antibiotics from their patients. Particularly in the US, the high cost of liability in the case of treatment failure may induce them to err on the side of caution — ie to use stronger and broader-spectrum drugs than may be necessary[2].

Strategies to increase appropriate use

Participative doctor feedback and multidisciplinary interventions have been found to increase the use of first-line antibiotics and reduce costs[3-5]. Studies have employed educational methods including regular mailings to front-line doctors containing personalized reports of antibiotic prescribing history (prepared confidentially) accompanied by guideline-based clinical messages. The cost of implementing such strategies is, however, considerable. Individualized feedback might be effective but possibly too costly to implement on a routine and widespread basis. (Such a programme may be more feasible in a managed-care or hospital setting where prescribing data are routinely collected.) Another strategy is rapid identification and susceptibility testing to aid appropriate antibiotic treatment selection[6].

The need for surveillance

Surveillance is a critical component in curtailing the development and persistence of microbial resistance. Information gathered from surveillance work must be timely, accurate and geographically relevant. On a local level, such information helps doctors to make clinical decisions and to update treatment recommendations. At a national and international level, this information guides the development of public health policies and allows the effectiveness of policy changes and intervention strategies to be assessed. Surveillance information helps to focus the research needed to estimate the cost of antibiotic resistance. For instance, the relationship between bacterial resistance and changes in antibiotic prescribing (dose–response rate) is currently unknown, but is known to be a critical parameter in the economic evaluation of resistance. Further research gathering surveillance data is needed to elucidate and define factors that are important for the emergence, persistence and transmission of antibiotic-resistant bacteria.

The cost of developing national and worldwide surveillance systems is uncertain. What is generally agreed, however, is that the design and maintenance of such a system would require large investments of both resources and coordination involving government agencies, health departments, independent laboratories and doctors. While the complexities and costs involved may be considerable, advances in information technology can help to minimize these barriers. Electronic laboratory-based reporting provides an efficient means of aggregating large amounts of data from independent laboratories and the Internet provides an up-to-the-minute, efficient means of disseminating information to doctors, policy makers and researchers.

A number of national and international efforts to collect data from microbiology laboratories are currently underway[7]. The WHO Collaborating Center for Surveillance of Antimicrobial Resistance is working with microbiology laboratories to facilitate the reporting of antibiotic susceptibility data, and the CDC collects data under the Active Bacterial Core Surveillance project for community infections. In the US, an interagency Task Force on Antimicrobial Resistance was created in 1999 to address antibiotic resistance. Surveillance for antibiotic resistance in bacteria that pose a public health threat has been identified as one of four major areas of focus.

Economic costs

Economic costs associated with antibiotic resistance can be attributed to at least three factors. Firstly, patients infected with resistant bacteria require longer hospitalization and face higher treatment costs than patients infected with drug-susceptible strains[8-11]. Secondly, society bears the cost associated with the higher risk of mortality in resistant infections[12]. Finally, the cost of introducing new antibiotics to replace old ineffective ones is high and increasing, and involves the commitment of resources that could be deployed to other public health research projects, such as developing new drugs for AIDS or cancer[13].

Resistance costs are rarely considered even in economic evaluations of antibiotic treatment alternatives because the uncertainty of the impact of current antibiotic use on future resistance. Although this uncertainty is considerable, some projections show that, even with conservative estimates, the cost of antibiotic resistance is high enough to influence cost–benefit decisions made at the individual prescription level[14]. Assuming that infections with resistant organisms can be fatal, and that resistance can persist for one year, the resultant annual cost of antibiotic resistance to society in general can range from $5 to $50 per individual prescription[15]. It appears that the cost of antibiotic resistance may be high enough to warrant inclusion in cost-effectiveness analyses of antibiotic treatments. At the very least, consideration of these costs should be included in a sensitivity analysis or a discussion of the results.

Assuming 150 million prescriptions are generated each year, the annual figure quoted most often for the economic impact of resistance in the US ranges from $350m to $35bn (at 1989 dollar rates)[15]. These estimates vary depending on:

- the rate at which resistance grows with respect to increasing antibiotic use
- the level of inappropriate antibiotic prescribing
- how long resistance persists in the bacterial population
- the discount rate used for future costs of resistance
- the probability that a patient will die following infection with a resistant pathogen.

A report by the Office of Technology Assessment to the US Congress estimated the annual cost associated with antibiotic resistance in hospitals to be at least $1.3bn (at 1992 dollar rates)[16]. This estimate only covered five classes of nosocomial infections from six different antibiotic-resistant bacteria. The Centers for Disease Control estimated that the cost of all hospital-acquired infections, including both antibiotic-resistant and antibiotic-susceptible strains in their figures was $4.5bn[16].

New antibiotics

The emergence of resistance has created new markets for antibiotics. The pharmaceutical industry can be a major player in the struggle against antibiotic resistance: producers can encourage appropriate antibiotic use, which will lengthen the market life of established drugs; in addition, drugs companies have a critical role in the development and production of novel antibiotics. In recognition of this role, national and international policy makers must consider economic incentives that influence the behaviour of the pharmaceutical industry. Under patent protection laws, pharmaceutical companies have a limited number of years to recoup R&D costs, so an economic incentive is present to push the drugs into wider applications. Aggressive marketing, including use of direct-to-consumer advertising, can increase antimicrobial resistance by encouraging inappropriate prescribing.

In response to these issues, several solutions have been suggested, including negotiated marketing agreements for antibiotics whose manufacturers would agree to restrict their marketing efforts in exchange for a longer patent protection period. Other possibilities include restructuring patent laws to allow renewed patent protection for drugs that have been previously patented but never entered the marketplace[16]. The expectation of a sufficient return on investments currently provides the incentive for the pharmaceutical industry to fund much of the new product research required, but the economic climate may always affect investment adversely. Currently, developing countries are most seriously affected by antibiotic resistance, compounded by factors such as poverty, overcrowding and unsanitary conditions[17]. The fact that these countries cannot afford to spend large amounts of money on antibiotics means pharmaceutical manufacturers have little economic incentive to develop new drugs for them. Even in developed countries where antibiotic resistance is a problem, the market may be relatively small when compared to the demand for treatments for such chronic illnesses as arthritis, diabetes or hypertension. Unless pharmaceutical companies can charge a high price for a new antibiotic product in a small market, their R&D dollars can be spent more profitably elsewhere. These economic factors affecting the motivation of pharmaceutical companies must be considered by national and international bodies who are examining policies to promote the development of new antibiotic products in the future.

Conclusions

The authors' recommendations include:
- Gathering current, accurate, geographically specific surveillance information on antibiotic resistance patterns.
- Funding epidemiological research to explore the relationship between changes in the prevalence of resistance and changes in the level of prescribing.
- Exploring the most effective methods of patient education about the risks associated with antibiotic misuse.
- Ensuring that policy makers consider the costs of inappropriate use when developing and evaluating prescribing policies and guidelines.
- Evaluating the cost-effectiveness of antibiotic treatment alternatives that explicitly consider the costs of antibiotic resistance.
- Undertaking the need for further research to understand and alter the treatment choices for patients and doctors, including the barriers imposed by health plans on prescribing.
- Research to explore the potential effects of altering patent protection laws for antibiotics.

References

1. Seppala H, Klaukka T, Vuopio-Varkila I et al. The effect of changes in the consumption of macrolide antibiotics on erythromycin resistance in group A streptococci in Finland. *N Engl J Med* 1998; **337**: 441-6.
2. Barden LS, Dowell SF, Schwartz B, Lackey C. Current attitudes regarding use of antimicrobial agents: results from physicians' and parents' focus group discussions. *Clin Pediatr* 1998; **37**: 665-72.
3. Zwar N, Wolk J, Gordon J, Sanson-Fisher R, Kehoe L. Influencing antibiotic prescribing in general practice: a trial of prescriber feedback and management guidelines. *Fam Pract* 1999; **16**: 495-500.
4. Hux JE, Melady MP, DeBoer D. Confidential prescriber feedback and education to improve antibiotic use in primary care: a controlled trial. *CMAJ* 1999; **161**: 388-92.
5. Gonzales R, Steiner JF, Lum A, Barrett PH Jr. Decreasing antibiotic use in ambulatory practice: impact of a multidimensional intervention on the treatment of uncomplicated acute bronchitis in adults. *JAMA* 1999; **281**: 1512-9.
6. Barenfanger J, Drake C, Kacich G. Clinical and financial benefits of rapid bacterial identification and antimicrobial susceptibility testing. *J Clin Microbiol* 1999; **37**: 1415-8.
7. Monnet DL. Toward multinational antimicrobial resistance surveillance systems in Europe. *Int J Antimicrob Agents* 2000; **15**: 91-101.
8. Holmberg SD, Solomon SL, Blake PA. Health and economic impacts of antimicrobial resistance. *Rev Infect Dis*. 1987; **9**: 1065-78.
9. Wakefield DS, Helms CM, Massanari RM, Mori M, Pfaller M. Cost of nosocomial infection: relative contributions of laboratory, antibiotic, and per diem costs in *Staphylococcus aureus* infections. *Am J Infect Control* 1988; **16**: 185-92.
10. Abramson MA, Sexton DJ. Nosocomial methicillin-resistant and methicillin-susceptible Staphylococcus aureus primary bacteremia: at what costs? *Infect Control Hosp Epidemiol* 1999; **20**: 408-11.
11. Rubin RJ, Harrington CA, Poon A et al. The economic impact of *Staphylococcus aureus* in New York city hospitals. *Emerg Infect Dis* 1999; **5**: 9-17.
12. Harthug S, Eide GE, Langeland N. Nosocomial outbreak of ampicillin resistant *Enterococcus faecium*: risk factors for infection and fatal outcome. *J Hosp Infect* 2000; **45**: 135-44.
13. Bax RP. Antibiotic resistance: a view from the pharmaceutical industry. *Clin Infect Dis* 1997; **24** (Suppl 1): S151-3.
14. Coast J, Smith RD, Millar MR. Superbugs: should antimicrobial resistance be included as a cost in economic evaluation. *Health Econ* 1996; **5**: 217-26.
15. Phelps CE. Bug/drug resistance: sometimes more is less. *Med Care* 1989; **27**: 194-203.
16. Office of Technology Assessment. Impact of antibiotic-resistant bacteria: A report to the U.S. Congress, 1995. OTA-H-629.
17. O'Brien TF. Global surveillance of antibiotic resistance. *N Engl J Med* 1992; **326**: 339-40.

The role of infectious agents in bronchitis

DR G. DOUGLAS CAMPBELL

PROFESSOR, LOUSIANA STATE UNIVERSITY MEDICAL CENTER, 1501 KINGS HIGHWAY, ROOM 6341, SHREVEPORT, LA 71103, USA

As defined by the American Thoracic Society, chronic bronchitis is recognized clinically when a patient has cough and sputum production for 3 months of the year over at least 2 consecutive years. The chronic production of sputum is a consequence of goblet cell hyperplasia and airway inflammation. An acute exacerbation of chronic bronchitis (AECB) is characterized by symptoms of increased dyspnea, increased sputum volume, and increased sputum purulence. The severity of the acute process can be graded by how many of these symptoms are present. In one study, Anthonisen and colleagues graded exacerbations as Type I if all three symptoms were present; Type II if only two symptoms were present; and Type III if only one symptom was present[1]. The efficacy of antibiotic therapy in AECB varied with the severity of the acute episode.

The frequency with which patients experience exacerbations is also an important factor which can be used to grade the severity of chronic bronchitis as a disease process. The distinction between simple and complicated chronic bronchitis is made by whether patients have four or more exacerbations per year. When sputum is cultured from a patient with chronic bronchitis, bacteria often are present, with nontypable *Haemophilus influenzae*, *Streptococcus pneumoniae*, and *Moraxella catarrhalis* being the most commonly recovered pathogens. The role of bacteria in actually causing an acute exacerbation is uncertain because the same organisms may be present when the patient is clinically stable or when the patient is having an acute exacerbation, reflecting the fact that these patients have chronic tracheobronchial colonization. Thus, the role of bacteria in patients with AECB is controversial, making the necessity of antibiotic therapy equally uncertain.

In interpretation and subsequent treatment, three questions arise. First, are these organisms actually present in the lower respiratory tract or do they simply represent contamination?

Second, if these organisms are present, do they affect lung function adversely? Third, is there evidence for the beneficial role of antimicrobial therapy in episodes of AECB? If bacteria are not important in the pathogenesis of chronic bronchitis and AECB, then antimicrobial therapy would not be expected to benefit the patient, but would add unnecessarily to the cost of therapy and might cause side-effects or even contribute to drug resistance. However, if bacteria are important in chronic bronchitis and AECB, then their role should be emphasized. In an earlier consensus report, the role of antimicrobial therapy was discussed only briefly and recommendations for antibiotic use and selection were limited[2].

Evidence that bacteria are present in the lower respiratory tract

There are several lines of evidence supporting the role of bacteria in AECB. First, bacteria can be recovered from the lower respiratory tract using protected specimen brushes via a fibre-optic bronchoscope (FOB-PSBs). In the past decade two major studies using FOB-PSBs have been performed to determine the incidence of bacteria in the lower respiratory tract. Monso et al performed FOB-PSBs on 40 stable outpatients with chronic bronchitis and 29 patients presenting with AECB[3]. Organisms were recovered from 13 individuals with stable bronchitis: 10 of these (25%) were recovered in concentrations of $\geq 10^3$ colony-forming units (CFUs) per ml, with *Haemophilus* spp (6) and *Streptococcus pneumoniae* (3) the most common isolates. Multiple isolates were recovered from three patients. In contrast, organisms were recovered from 19 of the 29 AECB patients: 15 of these samples (52%) were at concentrations of $\geq 10^3$ CFUs per ml, and the most common isolates were *Haemophilus* spp (10), *S. pneumoniae* (3), *M. catarrhalis* (2), and 10 different species of gram-negative bacilli. Fagon et al used FOB-PSBs to sample the lower respiratory tract of patients requiring mechanical ventilation due to respiratory failure because of AECB[4]. All patients were under the age of 85, had not received antimicrobial agents for at least 10 days, and had no pulmonary infiltrates on chest radiographs. Bacteria were found in half of the 54 patients sampled. In 24 of these patients the bacterial concentrations were $\geq 10^3$ CFU/ml, and *Haemophilus parainfluenzae* (11), *S. pneumoniae* (7), *H. influenzae* (5) and *M. catarrhalis* (3) were the most commonly isolated organisms.

Another study using FOB-PSBs looked for factors that might affect the spectra of potential pathogens. Soler et al carried out a comprehensive study of the upper and lower airways in 50 patients with severe AECB requiring mechanical ventilation[5]. In all, 34 potentially pathogenic micro-organisms from the lower respiratory tract were isolated, including *H. influenzae* (12 isolates), *Pseudomonas* spp (9 isolates), *S. pneumoniae* and *M. catarrhalis* (4 isolates each), as well as *Stenotrophomonas maltophilia* and *Enterobacter cloacae* (2 isolates each). The presence of

Pseudomonas spp and *Stenotrophomonas maltophilia* in such large numbers (28% of cases) was surprising, but not statistically significant — their occurrence was more common in the elderly (≥65 years) and among patients who had been hospitalized more than once in the past year. While bronchiectasis could be an explanation for the large number of *Pseudomonas* and *Stenotrophomonas* spp, clinical and radiographic evidence for bronchiectasis was not apparent.

Variations in the pathogen spectrum found in these studies were not completely addressed. The Soler study identified age and repeated hospitalization as factors[5], while a similar study looking at pathogens from the sputa of 112 AECB patients, found that the spectra of organisms changed as the forced expiratory volume in 1 second (FEV_1) declined[6]. *S. pneumoniae*, other gram-positive cocci, *H. influenzae* and *M. catarrhalis* were the most common isolates when FEV_1 was >1.5l, and *Enterobacteriaceae* spp and *Pseudomonas* spp were more common when the FEV_1 was <1.5l.

Additional evidence supporting a role for bacteria is the demonstration of the development of the bacteriocidal host immune response to the bacterium isolated from sputum samples. While earlier studies were unable to distinguish antibodies to antigenic determinants present on the bacterial surface[7], with the development of more advanced immunoassay techniques, specific bacteriocidal immune responses can now be detected to surface exposed antigens of the sputum bacterium recovered, but not to control organisms. To date, studies from patients have identified antibody responses to *M. catarrhalis*, *H. influenzae* and *H. parainfluenzae* from patients during an episode of AECB[8–10]. The elicitation of a such a human antibody response not only suggests that these organisms are present, but that the host recognizes them as foreign and is mounting an immune response. Serum bacteriocidal activity has been shown to be protective in otitis media, but no investigations of this protection have yet been reported for chronic bronchitis[11].

Additional evidence supporting the role of bacteria in AECB is the fact that antimicrobial therapy has been associated with a favourable clinical response among patients presenting with chronic bronchitis. Recent studies have shown that during bacteria-induced AECB there is an increase in interleuken-8, tumour necrosis factor-a, neutrophil elastase and myeloperoxidase markers, which indicate airway inflammation[12]. In addition, non-typeable *H. influenzae* has been shown not only to adhere to non-ciliated epithelial cells in the lower respiratory tract, but also to invade these cells so it can be found in the submucosa and interstitium[13,14].

These studies suggest that bacteria including *Haemophilus* spp, *M. catarrhalis* and *S. pneumoniae*, are present in the lower respiratory tract; their presence and concentration are more common during AECBs, but the spectrum of organisms recovered may vary based upon certain patient factors (age, FEV1, repeated hospitalizations). Based upon this information, antimicrobial therapy is expected to be beneficial, but the agents used should be carefully depending upon the most likely pathogens and the presence of antimicrobial resistance.

Does the presence of organisms in the lower respiratory tract affect lung function adversely?

An association between AECB and deteriorating lung function has been shown in one of four prospective studies[15]. Such longitudinal studies are difficult to perform, and a variety of contributing factors that can affect lung function may not be taken into account. Murphy and Sethi have proposed a 'vicious circle hypothesis' as the mechanism by which the bacteria may affect lower respiratory tract function[16]. Their proposal differs from the 'British hypothesis' by proposing that the primary initiating damage in chronic bronchitis results from factors including cigarette smoke and childhood respiratory diseases, with bacterial colonization playing an important but secondary role. Following initial damage to the lower respiratory tract, bacterial colonization occurs resulting in inflammation due to the presence of cell associated bacterial antigens (lipo-oligosaccharides from *H. influenzae* and *M. catarrhalis*, and capsular material from *S. pneumoniae*). The inflammatory response is a reaction to the secretion of bacterial products (eg lipo-oligosaccharides), elastase from recruited polymorphonuclear leucocytes, or the production of cytokines. These two arms result in continuing damage to airway epithelium and progression towards chronic obstructive pulmonary disease (COPD).

Antibiotic treatment of AECB

Studies performed since the 1950s to evaluate the role of antimicrobial agents in AECB were limited because of the size of the population sample, lack of a control arm and their use of antimicrobial agents that did not penetrate into the lower respiratory tract. The results therefore were conflicting.

The first large placebo controlled study into the role of antimicrobials in AECB was reported by Anthonisen *et al*[1] whose study enrolled 173 patients with AECB. Half of the patients received oral antimicrobial therapy (trimethoprim-sulfamethoxizole bid, or amoxicillin 250mg qid or doxycycline 200 mg initially and then 100 mg qid) and the other half received placebo. The severity of the patient's AECB was graded using 3 clinical indicators — increased dyspnea, increased sputum production and change in sputum purulence — and stratified into type 1, 2 or 3 AECB based upon 3, 2 or 1 clinical indicators respectively. Peak flow improved more rapidly in type 1 patients who were treated with antibiotics compared with type 1 placebo patients. No differences were noted between type 2 or type 3 patients receiving antibiotics compared with the corresponding control group.

More recently, a meta-analysis reported by Saint et al, incorporated all published studies of patients with AECB where there was a placebo control arm and showed a slight but significant improvement among patients with AECB receiving antimicrobial therapy[17]. The majority of studies included in this meta-analysis were published before 1980, enrolled small numbers of patients and did not stratify patients based upon the severity of AECB. Additionally, the antimicrobial choices used would not be considered first-line agents.

Allegra[18], presented a significant Italian study rarely cited in English literature, which selected the antibiotic most commonly used to treat AECB. In this double-blind, randomized, placebo-controlled, multi-centred trial, a short five day course of amoxicillin/clavulanate (7:1 combination) 1g twice-daily was compared to a placebo control in 369 patients. Therapy was initiated at an early stage in exacerbation and response was monitored using an integrated score derived from five factors (sputum production, sputum volume, sputum colour, temperature and dyspnea) which were graded for severity comparing the score at initiation of therapy to that at the end of the study. Results showed that the failure rate was significantly higher among controls than among the treated patients (49.7% vs. 13.6%, $p<0.001$), and both FEV1 and the integrated score improved more rapidly with antimicrobial therapy ($p<0.01$).

Studies to date suggest that antimicrobial therapy is associated with rapid improvement in AECB, but these investigations have not addressed whether or not antimicrobial therapy has a long-term effect on the recurrence of AECB. Anzueto reported a recent retrospective study of 173 outpatients who experienced 362 episodes of AECB and were over an 18-month period[19]. No antimicrobial therapy was initiated in 92 cases. Patients were stratified by exacerbation type, severity of COPD (by baseline FEV_1), the presence of comorbidities and other demographic factors The relapse rate was significantly higher among the non-treated group with 32% requiring a return visit compared to only 19% ($p<0.001$) among the treated group. Relapse rates were associated with smoking, coronary artery disease and the lack of antimicrobial therapy rather than the severity of the underlying disease or intensity of AECB. However, not all antimicrobial agents were equally effective, as patients treated with amoxicillin had a higher relapse rate than those receiving other antimicrobial therapy.

The Anzueto study corroborates the earlier work of Ball[20] which showed that cardiopulmonary disease was a risk factor for a return doctor's visit, and also a study by Grossman that recognized that the time between AECB episodes was influenced by the antibiotic chosen[21]. In the Grossman study, 240 patients with frequent type 1 or 2 AECB were studied over 12 months. Patients were randomized to receive either ciprofloxacin or the standard antibiotic therapy selected by the primary care physician, which could also be ciprofloxacin. Patients who received ciprofloxacin experienced a longer symptom free interval before their next AECB episode, and while costs were not significantly different between the two arms, trends in outcomes and all quality of life measures favoured ciprofloxacin.

Conclusions

The studies reported to date support four points:
- bacteria are common in the lower respiratory tract of chronic bronchitis patients especially during episodes of AECB
- bacteria incite a host response as well as releasing proteins which may damage the lower respiratory tract
- antimicrobial therapy is associated with improved response
- certain antimicrobial agents produce a longer symptom free interval.

Bronchitis is a common illness and antibiotic agents are not always appropriate for use because of their cost, caution over the development of drug resistance or lack of evidence to support efficacy. Antimicrobial agents should not be given to patients with otherwise normal respiratory function, since in this setting, pollutants and respiratory viruses are by far the most common causes of ill health and such episodes usually resolve on their own without intervention.

As lung function deteriorates, bacterial causes are often implicated in lung difficulties, but since bronchitis is a mucosal infection, antimicrobial agents are not always advisable because indiscriminate use may assist the development of antibiotic resistance. While a clear association between bacteria and AECB has yet to be definitively proven[22], clinical studies point to the beneficial effect of antibiotic therapy among type 1 and 2 AECB patients. Only if AECB is prolonged should antimicrobial agents be considered to reduce AECB-related morbidity, prevent the need for hospitalization, and limit the inflammatory response from causing further damage to the lower respiratory tract.

Drug choice should be based upon patient-related factors (such as age, number of AECBs per year, the patient's baseline FEV1) alongside the most likely target pathogen with an appreciation of existing antimicrobial resistance. New broad-spectrum antibiotics are able to penetrate the lower respiratory tract in high concentrations with a prolonged post-antibiotic effect and longer infection-free intervals. Potentially this should mean treatment can not only reduce the number of AECB episodes but also act prophylactically to prevent further attacks.

References

1. Antonisen NR, Manfreda J, Warren W et al. Antibiotic therapy in exacerbations of chronic obstructive pulmonary disease. Ann Intern Med 1987; **106**: 196-204.
2. Anonymous Standards for the diagnosis and care of patients with chronic obstructive pulmonary disease. American Thoracic Society. Am J Respir Crit Care Med 1995 ; **152**: s77–121.
3. Monso E, Ruiz J, Rosell A et al. Bacterial infection in chronic obstructive pulmonary disease. A study of stable and exacerbated outpatients using the protected specimen brush. Am J Respir Crit Care Med 1995; **152**:1316-20.
4. Fagon J, Chastre J, Trouillet JL et al. Characterization of distal bronchial microflora during acute exacerbation of chronic bronchitis. Am Rev Respir Dis 1990; **142**:1004-8.
5. Soler N, Torres A, Ewig S, Gonzalez J, Celis R, El-Ebiary M, Hernandez C, Rodriguez-Roisin R. Bronchial microbial patterns in severe exacerbations of chronic obstructive pulmonary disease (COPD) requiring mechanical ventilation. Am J Respir Crit Care Med 1998; **157**:1498-1505.
6. Eller J, Ede A, Schaberg T et al. Infective exacerbations of chronic bronchitis: relation between bacteriologic etiology and lung function. Chest 1998; **113**: 1542–8.
7. Musher DM, Kubitschek KR, Crennan J, Baugh RE. Pneumonia and acute febrile tracheobronchitis due to Haemophilus influenzae. Ann Intern Med 1983; **99**: 444–50.
8. Murphy TF, Kirkkham C, DeNardin E, Sethi S. Analysis of antigenic structure and human immune response to outer membrane protein CD of Moraxella catarrhalis. Infect Immun 1999; **67**: 4578–85.
9. Yi K, Sethi S, Murphy TF. Human immune response to nontypable Haemophilus influenzae in chronic bronchitis. J Infect Dis 1997; **176**: 1247–52.
10. Mitchell JL, Hill SL. Immune response to Haemophilus parainfluenzae in patients with chronic obstructive lung disease. Clin Diagn Lab Immunol 2000; **7**: 25–30.
11. Fjaden H, Bernstein J, Brodsky L et al. Otitis media in children. I. The systemic immune response to nontypable Haemophilus influenzae. J Infect Dis 1989; **160**: 999–1004.
12. Sethi S, Muscarella K, Evans N et al. Comparison of airway inflammation in acute bacterial and non-bacterial exacerbations of COPD. Am J Respir Crit Care Med 1999; **159**: A822.
13. Moller LVM, Tmens W, van der Bi W et al. Haemophilus influenzae in lung explants of patients with end-stage pulmonary disease. Am J Respir Crit Care Med 1998; **157**: 950–6.
14. Ketterer MR, Shao JQ, Hornic DB et al. Infection of primary human bronchial epithelial cells by Haemophilus influenzae; macropinocytosis as a mechanism of epithelial cell entry. Infect Immun 1999; **67**: 4161–70.
15. Wilson R. The role of infection in COPD. Chest 1998; **113**: 242s–8.
16. Murphy TF, Sethi S. Bacterial infection in chronic obstructive pulmonary disease. Am Rev Respir Dis 1992; **146**: 1067–83.
17. Saint S, Bent S, Vittinghoff E, Grady D. Antibiotics in chronic obstructive pulmonary disease exacerbations: a meta-analysis. JAMA 1995; **273**: 957–60.
18. Allegra L, Grassi C, Grossi E. The role of antibiotics in the treatment of chronic bronchitis exacerbations: follow-up of a multicenter study. Ital J Dis Chest 1991; **45**: 138–45.
19. Adams SG, Melo J, Luther M, Anzueto A. Antibiotics are associated with lower relapse rates in outpatients with acute exacerbations of COPD. Chest 2000; **117**: 1345–52.
20. Ball P, Harris JM, Lowson D, Tillotson G, Wilson R. Acute infective exacerbations of chronic bronchitis. Q J Med 1995; **88**: 61-8.
21. Grossman R, Mukherjee J, Vaughan D et al. A 1-year community-based health economic study of ciprofloxacin vs. usual antibiotic treatment in acute exacerbations of chronic bronchitis: the Canadian Ciprofloxacin Health Economic Study Group. Chest 1998; **113**: 131–41.
22. Murphy TF, Sethi S, Niederman MS. The role of bacteria in exacerbations of COPD. A constructive view. Chest 2000; **118**: 193–203.

The role of the pharmaceutical industry in fostering the appropriate use of antibiotics

MS RITA KUNZ

ASSOCIATE DIRECTOR GLOBAL SCIENTIFIC AFFAIRS, BAYER AG, BUSINESS GROUP PHARMA,
42096 WUPPERTAL, GERMANY

There is a need for a major change in how the pharmaceutical industry addresses the growing problem of microbial resistance to antibiotics. For far too long the pharmaceutical industry has developed new agents in a microbe-by-microbe approach, but essentially struggling to create new antibiotics to overcome the various bacteria that have overcome the traditional first-line agents as opposed to addressing the larger issue of microbial resistance.

Within this paper we address the important topic of the role of the pharmaceutical industry in fostering and encouraging the appropriate use of antibiotics from both the prescriber and patient perspectives as that is probably the most important way to successfully address the problem of antimicrobial resistance.

Bayer consider the top priority to be the maintenance of the efficacy of antibiotic classes for as long as possible. Antibiotics are not a renewable resource. Only one new class of antibacterial, oxazolidinones, has been developed in the last 25 years. The other 'new' antibiotics have been refinements and chemical extensions of existing classes. It is imperative that we encourage physicians to use antibiotics only when they maximize therapeutic outcome, minimize resistance development, and reduce the economic and human burdens of infection. It is only through the *appropriate use* of antibiotics these goals can be achieved.

Clearly we do not wish to suggest that the pharmaceutical industry should stop actively marketing antibiotics to physicians and other healthcare professionals. Obviously, they want practitioners to know about their latest advances in drug development, indeed many physicians receive much of their continuing education from the industry. However, the pharmaceutical industry needs to analyze their promotional and educational materials carefully to make sure that they are fostering the *appropriate use* of these drugs.

In a recent publication on infectious disease and antimicrobial resistance[1], the World Health Organization (WHO) report stated that "the most effective strategy against antimicrobial resistance is to get the job done right the first time to defeat resistance before it starts". The report advocates effective therapy, delivered effectively. The pharmaceutical industry must play its part to encourage physicians to use an effective and *appropriate* antibiotic. It should only be used when an antibiotic is really necessary.

The pharmaceutical industry should be encouraging physicians to consider the appropriate antibiotic as the first line of attack on possible-bacterial infection. Physicians should not take the approach of using low dose, long-term therapy with an antibiotic that may not provide adequate coverage of the pathogen, which is an ideal milieu for antibiotic resistance proliferation. This approach will not help the patient and it will not help curb resistance. Instead, it may make the resistance problem worse, leave the patient sicker for longer, and increase the cost of health care.

We need to re-think the overall approach that the pharmaceutical industry takes with regard to antibiotic development and use. At Bayer, we would like to suggest:

- Working with regulatory authorities to achieve labeling for antibiotics that recommends using the highest, safe dose for a shorter duration and thus improving compliance and preventing patients from curtailing therapy when they feel better
- Educating patients not to expect a prescription for antibiotics every time they have an infection but when they do get one, to take the medication as directed
- Encourage physicians to evaluate whether or not a patient really needs a course of antibiotics or whether some other treatment is more appropriate
- Improving understanding of the pharmacokinetics and phamacodynamics of antibiotics in humans and teaching physicians and other healthcare workers how to use antibiotics to optimal effect by selecting the right drug for the right disease at the right dose for the right duration.

The pharmaceutical industry is adopting some of these approaches and is keen to partner with health care authorities and academic groups in non-promotional ways to improve the current situation. It is in the long-term interest of the Industry.

We believe that the key to preventing resistance lies in giving a patient an antibiotic **only** when it is needed; in using antibiotics that are the **most appropriate**, rather than the cheapest; and in thoughtfully selecting the **most pharmacodynamically active** antibiotic for the **shortest duration** that is safe and will eradicate **the microbes faster**, preventing them from building up resistance. This will cure the patient sooner, and will save society money by reducing the overall cost of treatment and by getting the patient back to work sooner. That is why fostering the *appropriate* use of antibiotics and selecting the appropriate product for the first course of antibiotic therapy is of high importance.

This approach is not exclusive to human use. In 1998 the Bayer Animal Health Division issued one of the first set of guidelines for prudent use of antimicrobials in food producing animals[2]. The revised and extended guidelines on the use of fluoroquinolones in veterinary medicine were released in April 1999 and specifically addressed the use of the fluoroquinolones in veterinary medicine[3]. These guidelines were created to ensure that fluoroquinolones are used only for therapy in severe bacterial infections after microbial culture and susceptibility testing. Bayer is now actively implementing these guidelines world wide.

Encouraging the *appropriate* use of antibiotics is a 'win-win' proposition. It will help in the battle against disease because it will reduce bacterial resistance. It will help patients because the treatments they receive will be more effective; it will help physicians, because it will *assist* them to treat more patients successfully, and it will help industry, because it will ensure that we continue to have effective antibiotics to produce.

If fossil fuels are in danger of being used up, so may be antibiotics. The development of policies for antibiotic use should ensure that these agents which were genuine "wonder-drugs" will be available for our grandchildren. Bayer's scientific and clinical experts want to assume an important role in the efforts essential to contain the development of antibacterial resistance. There are three priorities:

1) To continue research and development to discover efficacious innovative antibiotics. Introduction of novel classes of antibacterial agents in the therapy of infectious diseases may be an efficient way to overcome existing problems;
2) To research the mechanisms, epidemiology and driving factors of microbial resistance. Investment will establish a clearer understanding of resistance. These results will allow the proper development of new antibacterial agents.
3) To provide guidance about how to maintain the continued value of current antibiotics. Educational initiatives for both health professionals (human and veterinary) and the general public have to address both the appropriate use of antibiotics, and using the appropriate antibiotic.

To preserve the effectiveness of antibiotics demands that we explain to all stakeholders the importance of implementing **appropriate antibiotic use.**

References

1. World Health Organization. *Overcoming Antimicrobial Resistance. World Health Report on Infectious Diseases 2000.* http://www.who.int/infectious-disease-report/2000/other_versions/index-rpt2000_text.html (Last accessed 15 August 2001).

2. Appropriate use of antimicrobials in animals. Leverkusen: Bayer AG, 1998.

3. Appropriate use of quinolones in food-producing animals. Leverkusen: Bayer AG, 1999.

NOTES

NOTES